The Arduous Touch

with warm regards,
Ruth Purtilo
4/28/1999

4/28/99
Best wishes
Kate Brown

Thank you
for your
interest in
our stories.
Amy Haddad
4/28/99

That we might
always remember the
voice of the voiceless
Frankly,
Claudia

The Ardous Touch

Women's Voices in Health Care

edited by Amy Marie Haddad and Kate H. Brown

NotaBell Books

An imprint of
Purdue University Press
West Lafayette, Indiana

∞ The paper used in this book meets the minimum requirements of
American National Standard for Information Sciences—Permanence of
Paper for Printed Library Materials, ANSI Z39.48-1992.

Printed in the United States of America

Library of Congress Cataloging-in-Publication Data

The arduous touch : voices of women in health care / edited by Amy Marie
    Haddad and Kate H. Brown.
        p.   cm.
    ISBN 1-55753-154-4 (alk. paper)
    1. Medical personnel, Writings of, American.   2. Medical personnel
and patient—United States—Literary collections.   3. Women in medicine—United States—Literary collections.   4. American literature—
Women authors.   5. American literature—20th century.   I. Haddad, Amy
Marie.   II. Brown, Kate H., 1950– .
PS508.M35A73 1999
810.8'09287'08861—dc21   98-55266
                                                                        CIP

Contents

Acknowledgments

Many thanks are due many creative people for their support of our efforts to bring these writings to you, our readers. Deep appreciation is extended to the Nebraska Humanities Council and the Creighton University Center for Health Policy and Ethics for their funding of "Logic of the Psyche: Health Care Ethics and Humanities," the writing group project in 1993–94 that led to this book. We are especially grateful to our contributors for their courage to do what they do every day in health care. They care wholeheartedly, even when it means that their whole hearts are broken for time to time. Special thanks also to our writing guides at the University of Nebraska, Lincoln: Judith Leven, Barbara DiBernard, Karen Foster, Kim Ports, Judith Slater, and Anne Whitney. In addition, we appreciated the feedback and encouragement we received for our colleagues at the Hiram College Center for Literature and Medicine. For their help with transforming our manuscript into a book, we thank Anne Keefe and Pat Hilliard-Barry. Many thanks also to Thomas Bacher and Margaret Hunt at the Purdue University Press for their encouragement and warm reception of this collection.

Introduction

Holding a dead baby. Standing up to a supervisor. Washing a bedridden patient's hair. Talking past and through one another in a case conference. Smoothing a sheet over a patient's disintegrating body. Firing a longtime friend and coworker.

These are some of the moments for ethical reflection portrayed in this anthology by women in health care. The authors write about the frustrations, fear, anger, hope, friendship, and awe they have felt working with patients of all ages and families in a variety of settings.

Literature can be a rich source of guidance to help with contemporary ethical dilemmas facing health care professionals and patients. Poems and stories can help us to identify moral problems, promote empathy, and tolerate ambiguity in health and illness. The depth and detail within stories and poems allow readers to experience the contradictory feelings, complex relationships, and situational messiness that characterize ethical quandaries in actual practice. These works by women in health care contribute to our understanding by introducing characters who struggle with illness and aging or who try to make sense of their own feelings in the face of pain and mortality. Who better to capture the essence of this complexity than people working directly in it?

This anthology is divided into three parts, reflecting three major themes in feminist perspectives in ethics: *power and powerlessness, vulnerability and voice, connection and disconnection.* The works included in the section on power and powerlessness bring to light the hidden issues of inequities of power in health care. Ironically, not only do patients feel powerless, but often caregivers do too. In the section on vulnerability and voice, the authors express the inability to be heard in the health care system. Related to issues of power and powerlessness, some of the works explore the experience of losing one's voice, either due to disease, mental illness, or social coercion. Other works explore attempts to find a voice that can be heard over the cacophony that accompanies ethical deliberation. The writings in the section dealing with connection and disconnection focus on the myriad relationships that are established, nurtured, and broken in the chaotic, impersonal environment of health care. These poems and stories reflect the place where professionals and patients meet and recognize shared joys and tragedies. They also explore the perhaps unbridgeable distances between the caregiver and cared-for.

Most of the works were written by women who participated in a year-long writing group cosponsored by the Nebraska Humanities Council and the Creighton University Center for Health Policy and Ethics. Additional contributions came from women health professionals throughout the United States. We are nurses, physicians, therapists, administrators, researchers, emergency room technicians, counselors, and social workers. Some have previously published. All share a passion for expressing their values, experiences, and ethical beliefs through creative writing. We invite our readers to use the stories and poems in this anthology to help them sort through their own personal questions and reflections about ethical issues in their lives.

*Power
and
Powerlessness*

FIRST BIRTH

Amy Haddad

Bent legs strapped snugly to stirrups,
Wrists restrained to the sides of the cart,

Barely covered by a surgical drape,
her legs, genitals, yellow with betadine,
exposed to the room,
she struggles and strains to free herself.

She is wet with sweat and she screams,
rhythmically, with each contraction.

She mutters, then shouts, "Please stop!
Get the fuck off me! It hurts! God, it hurts!
Stop it, please stop!"

The obstetrician says,
"You should have said that nine months ago."
The resident chuckles.

The nurse brushes the woman's damp hair back
and whispers into her ear,
"Shh, shh, shh, it's almost over, honey,"
but she struggles even harder at her restraints.

The obstetrician and resident play catch
with a small towel
back and forth over her.

She holds her breath and grunts,
bearing down,
giving birth.

"Finally," the obstetrician huffs.
The room is quiet now
until the baby cries.

She falls back on the table,
spent and drenched.

The nurse brushes the woman's damp hair back
and whispers into her ear,
"It's over, honey. You had a baby.
A baby girl."

BLAME PLACING

Amy Haddad

Surgical instruments clink against each other as
they drop onto the sterile cloth.

Holding the scalpel in his gloved hand like a baton,
poised above the blackened crust
that had once been her big toe—
tap, tap, tap, ready, begin.
The audience of attentive students circles
round the maestro.

I reach for the patient's hand,
hold it in both of mine.

He begins cutting away the decayed part of her toe
with constant clinical patter.

At first she does not flinch,
her hand still in mine.
Suddenly she squeezes my hands,
bites her bottom lip,
inhales sharply,
holds her breath against the pain.

Pleased, he pronounces, "Now we're getting somewhere.
See how it bleeds. That's a good sign."

I whisper close to her ear,
"Try and take a deep breath.
It will help ease the pain."
The smallest cry of anguish escapes as she exhales.
She turns crimson with shame.

The performance interrupted,
he hisses, "Let go of her hand."
She grabs me tighter.
He looks up, drops the scalpel,
snaps off both sterile gloves.
"I want to see you in the hall. Now."
Extracting my hands from hers,
I follow him out of the room.

Each word punctuated with a jab to my chest,
just above my name tag,
"When I tell you to let go of my patient, do it."
He pivots to leave,
then not quite finished, he turns back,
face so close to mine I feel his breath,
"You made things worse by babying her."
Students in tow, he leaves.

I return to dress her bloody foot.
Tears linger in the corner of her eyes,
"I'm sorry I got you in trouble," she says.

AS ORDERED

Ruth Ann Vogel

That Sunday afternoon
the Pediatric Ward
seemed even lighter
with the sun shining
through the west windows,
splashing on white walls,
white iron beds
and spreads of ribbed muslin.

Coming on duty at 3 P.M.
in fresh apron and cap,
like most students,
I was excited to work in Pediatrics again.

My assignment:
  Patient, female, age 11, Winnebago
  Prep. (shave entire scalp)
  Surgery in A.M.

My patient, Sunflower, sat erect,
legs crossed, on her white spread
a pre-teen with smooth, amber skin,
brushing her raven hair, shiny and thick
long and straight as a plumb line,
hiding most of her hospital gown.

Screening her area with a tri-frame
of more bleached muslin,
I introduced myself
while silently praying
for an act of nature, a fire,

an earthquake,
or a ram in a burning bush,
in the next five minutes.

Anything to prevent this order
from being carried out
or that I could trade places
with this beautiful child
who sat motionless, alone
silent as a dove.

Prepare her, I thought. Tell her,
"The surgeon will remove a plug
from the skull, like a watermelon,
to see if it is pink inside."

I told her, "The doctor wants me
to cut your hair. It will grow back."

She saw my scissors and my tears.
She was very brave.
I parted her hair,
wove two thick braids,
tied and cut them
and gave them to her to hold.

I cropped her hair close to the scalp,
shaved her head, using lather
and a double-edged razor,
and shaved again.
Finally, it was finished.

She reached with both hands
clutching her bald head.
Courage gave way to sobbing.
We cried together.

In the A.M., I met the gurney in the hall.
She was being carted off to surgery.
She never returned.
Diagnosis: T.B. of the brain
And I—
I write that I might wash away the pain.

PROCEDURES

Kim Dayton

"It's kind of like a fish out of water," said the doctor, who was not really a doctor yet.

"What do you mean, a fish?" I asked.

"Well, what I mean is, do you know how a fish can't breathe when it's out of the water? Well, the baby has a similar problem."

"But the other doctor said it was breathing," I said, "and the nurse also said that the baby was breathing."

"Yes, but you see, these babies, I mean these tiny ones like yours, sometimes they can breathe just fine for a while, but then after a while they just get tired and then we have to help them."

"How do you help them?"

"Well, we have a device that helps them, just for a while, until the baby is able to breathe on her own."

"Why are you telling me this?"

"It's just that I didn't want you to be alarmed when you saw the baby."

"What do you mean, alarmed?"

"Well, the baby has some tubes and things."

"You mean an IV? I'm not stupid, you know."

"No, I don't mean the IV, Mrs. Colson, the baby still has the IV," said the doctor, and he tapped his pencil on the table, "but you see, now the baby has some additional tubes."

"Where are the tubes?"

"Well, we have to put the tubes in the baby's mouth, I mean, down the baby's throat into her lungs."

"Can I see the baby?"

"Yes, eventually of course, but I'm afraid you will not be able to hold the baby. That is part of our standard nursery procedure."

Then the nurse came over and said, "Is this Mom?"

I'm Mom, yes, I guess I'm Mom. So I said, "I'm Mom."

"Well, Mom, we know that this is very scary for you, but your baby is getting the best of care, and I think that it might be best if you just try to get some rest. Do you plan to pump?"

"What do you mean, do I plan to pump?"

"Well, what I mean is, were you planning to breast feed the baby?"

And I said, "I guess; I hadn't really thought about it much."

"Well, you know, breast milk is really best for babies, especially the very tiny ones like yours, and if you would like, we can show you the procedure. Now, I must emphasize that you must pump very regularly, I mean, every four hours at least, day and night."

"Wait a minute, just how long is the baby going to be here?"

The nurse looked at the other one, the doctor, who was not really a doctor yet, and said, "Well, I think she will probably be here for quite a while."

Then the doctor, who was not really a doctor yet, said, "Have you gone down to the billing office?"

And I said, "I think that's already taken care of."

"Well, it says here on the chart that you need to be seen in billing, so perhaps you should go down there now."

"But when will I get to see the baby?"

And the nurse said, "They are doing some procedures right now, so it will be a while, so why don't you just go on down to billing, and then go get some rest, and then perhaps everything will be ready and you can see the baby."

"Procedures? What do you mean, procedures?"

"Did anyone show you the parents' sleeping room?"

And I said, "Yes."

Then the doctor said, "Where is Dad?" and I just looked at him.

Then later, after I had rested, and while I was scrubbing for two minutes like the sign said, a different nurse came over and said, "Mrs. Colson?"

And I said, "Yes."

And she said, "I'm afraid you can't go in just now."

"Why not?"

"Well, it's time for rounds."

"Rounds?"

"That's when the doctors and the residents observe and discuss the babies."

And I asked, "How long does that take?"

And she said, "It depends."

So I took the chance and went and drank coffee in the cafeteria, and ate some Doritos, and then I went back upstairs. And a woman came over and she said, "Are you Mrs. Colson?"

And I said, "Yes."

"Well, my name is Miss Antonio and I'm the social worker."

"I'm not on welfare, you know."

"No, you see, I am the hospital social worker," said Antonio, and she patted my hand, "I'm here to help you in any way I can."

"Well then," I said, "maybe you can help me see my baby."

And she said, "Well, why don't I check." So she left and then she came back and she said, "Well, you can't go in right now."

"Why not?"

"They are changing shifts and no one can come in while they are changing shifts."

And I said, "Can I go in after that?"

She looked at her watch and said, "Probably."

And then she gave me a book and said, "Why don't you read this, it will tell you everything you need to know." So I opened the book and tried to read, but then I stopped trying to read, and looked at the pictures, and then I fell asleep.

When I woke up, it was dark outside and quiet in the parents' waiting room. So I went over to the window and I said to the girl there, who was not a nurse, "Can I go in now?" and right then a nurse looked up through the glass and she came through the door.

And she said, "Why don't you go sit in the parents' waiting room? The doctor needs to speak to you."

"Is there something wrong with my baby?"

"The doctor needs to talk to you."

So I sat and sat, and that same nurse came out for a while and said, "He will be with you soon." And after a long time I got very thirsty, but I was afraid to leave.

And then finally the doctor, who was not really a doctor yet, came out and said, "Mrs. Colson?"

And I said, "Goddammit, my name is not *Mrs.* Colson!"

"I'm sorry, *Miss* Colson, we had a minor problem, but it is all taken care of and the baby is doing just fine now."

"What kind of problem?"

"Well, do you remember earlier when I told you about the tube?"

"You mean the breathing tube?"

And he said, "Yes, well, sometimes these tubes malfunction."

"What do you mean, malfunction?" I asked.

"Well, they can get plugged up and when that happens there is a problem."

And I said, "Is my baby dead?".

"No, Mrs. Colson, of course not, but she did have what we call a code."

"What do you mean, a code?"

"Well, she stopped breathing and her heart stopped, but we were able to use some medication, and some procedures, and her heart started up again."

"Can I see her now?"

"Mrs. Colson, this incident was very stressful for her and so perhaps it would be best to wait for a while longer. Have you pumped recently?"

So I used the electric machine and I pumped again, and then I scrubbed again, and then I went over to the window and I said, "Could I please see my baby now?"

And the nurse said, "Please put on the gown. Do you know where your baby is?"

And I said, "No."

"What is your baby's name?"

And I said, "Star."

"Well, I don't think we have a baby named Star in here. Are you certain you are in the right place?"

And I said, "Goddammit, I want to see my baby."

And she called out, "Dr. Franklin, I need you over here for a minute. Mrs. Star is a little confused."

Then the woman doctor, whose name was Franklin, looked over and said, "That's Mrs. Colson."

And the nurse said, "Oh, Colson. Why did you say your name was Star?"

"I didn't say my name was Star. I said my baby's name was Star."

And the nurse looked at me, and then at her list, and then at me again, and said, "She's in A."

So then the doctor asked, "Who has the Colson baby?"

And a fat nurse said, "I do," and then, "Are you Mom?"

And I said, "I'm Mom, but I don't feel like a mom because my baby is two days old and I've never seen her."

So the fat nurse took me over to the incubator and the baby was in there and I guess it was my baby because the incubator said Baby Girl Colson. But when I looked at the baby, I could think only about a fish out of water and how the baby looked like a fish. Except that she was not flopping like a fish out of water would be, in fact she was not moving at all, and I said, "I think she's dead, she's not moving at all."

And the fat nurse said, "No, dear, she's not dead, she's paralyzed."

"My God, no one told me she was paralyzed."

"No, I mean we gave her something to paralyze her."

And I asked, "Why?"

And the fat nurse sighed and said, "Because she was fighting the vent."

"What does that mean, fighting the vent?"

"It means she was trying to breath."

"But I thought she was supposed to breathe."

"Not while she's on the vent."

"Why doesn't she have any fingernails?"

And the nurse looked at her clipboard and wrote something and said, "She will get fingernails when she is bigger. Have you pumped recently?"

And I said, "I will, but right now I would like to look at my baby," and so I did. I looked at my baby called Baby Girl Colson on the incubator, but named Star by me because she was supposed to be the light of my life, and I cried.

And a nurse, who was not my baby's nurse but another baby's nurse, came over and said, "Is something wrong?"

And I said, "No."

Then the fat nurse said, "Mrs. Colson, you will need to leave for a while because we need to do some procedures."

"What kind of procedures?" I asked.

"Standard procedures."

"Like what?"

And she said, "Well, we have to draw some blood, and we have to suction, and weigh her, and so on, and I think it would be best if you just stepped out."

So I stepped out, but now that I knew where my baby was, I watched through the window and I saw the nurse take her out of her incubator and put her on a scale. And the procedures took quite a while and then right after the nurse finished the procedures, the doctors came by, doing their rounds, I guess. I was standing by the window, but then I felt very faint and so I went to the parents' room to sit down and a man came by and said, "Hi, my name is Reverend Duke. I'm the hospital chaplain."

And I said, "Well, thank you, but I'm not a Catholic."

And he said, "Why, that's quite all right because I'm non-denominational and I'm here to help you in any way I can."

"Well then, maybe you could pray for my baby, Baby Girl Colson."

And he said, "Why, certainly I will." And he left. And then I went to the cafeteria and I had some scrambled eggs because by now it was breakfast time and my baby was three days old.

Then I went back upstairs, and pumped again, and scrubbed

again, and then went in to look at my baby in the incubator. There was a new, thin nurse standing there and she asked, "Are you Mom?"

And I said, "So they tell me."

"Well Mom, she is a beautiful baby."

"Thank you, but I think she looks a little bit like a fish."

And the nurse said, "I've never heard that one before, most people think they look like little old men," and she laughed. And right then an alarm started ringing and she pushed a button on a machine and it stopped.

And I said, "What's that?"

And she said, "Oh nothing, it's not picking up."

And I said, "Well, what's it for?"

"It tells us about her oxygen level."

"Is there some problem with her oxygen level?"

"Well, it dropped, but it's coming up now, see the numbers?"

And I did see that the numbers were going up and then they stopped. And I asked, "Is she OK now?"

And the nurse said, "She's just fine."

So I asked, "Can I hold her?"

"Oh no, I'm sorry, but our procedure doesn't allow you to hold her while she's on the vent."

"Yesterday the nurse was holding her to weigh her."

And the thin nurse said, "Well, yes, but weighing is important and we have to hold her to weigh her."

And I said, "Oh."

Then I sat for quite a while watching my baby, who was no longer paralyzed, but moving sometimes, and then I said to the thin nurse, "When do you feed her?"

And the thin nurse said, "Well, right now we are feeding her with this IV, but pretty soon, in a few days I would think, we will begin to feed her orally. Have you pumped recently?"

And I said, "Well, maybe I'd better go do that."

And the thin nurse asked, "Do you have anyone here with you?"

And I asked, "What do you mean?"

"I mean a family member or a friend."

And I said, "My mom threw me out."

"Well, I think you need to go home and get some rest."

"I think I'll just stay here a while longer."

And while I was sitting there, a lab person came up with some results, and the nurse looked at the results, and then said to another nurse, "I need to find Dr. Franklin. Can you watch my baby?"

And I said, "It's my baby."

And the nurse left and then came back with Dr. Franklin and Dr. Franklin said, "Put in a line."

And the nurse said, "Mrs. Colson, you will have to leave now."

"What's wrong?"

And Dr. Franklin said, "The baby is septic."

And I asked, "What does that mean, septic?"

And the thin nurse said, "She has an infection."

And I said, "Can't you give her something?"

"Of course we will. Why don't you leave now."

I said, "I'd like to stay, please."

"No, I'm sorry, you can't."

So I left and waited for a long time and then I eventually fell asleep.

Then when I woke up, I went to the window, but I couldn't see my baby because there were several doctors and nurses around the incubator. So I started to scrub, but then a nurse came through the door and said, "Mrs. Colson," and she laid her hand on my arm.

And I said, "What?"

And she said, "I'm so sorry."

And I said, "What?"

And she said, "Your baby died."

And I said, "Oh no," or maybe I said, "Oh my God," or "Star," or maybe it was something else.

And the doctor, who was not a doctor yet, and the doctor named Franklin came through the door then and Dr. Franklin said, "Mrs. Colson, we did everything we could. She just wasn't strong enough."

And the doctor, who was not a doctor, said, "She was septic."

And I looked at him and said, "Yes, I know."

Then a new and different nurse came through the door and asked, "Would you like to hold the baby?"

So finally I got to hold the baby, Baby Girl Colson, Star Maria Colson, who did not look to me like a fish anymore at all and who died because, even though she was strong enough to fight the vent, she just wasn't strong enough. And I thought about the room where we would have lived, and my cat, and the little booties that I bought when I first knew, and how he looked when I told him.

And I decided that next time I would do what my mom said to and just go have a procedure.

THE PATIENT CARE CONFERENCE
Susan Ogborn

"I just want them to show some respect for me . . . to understand that I'm her mother."

"What she has to understand is these doctors are busy; they can't stand around waiting for her to come, and besides, she doesn't always understand anyway."

"I'm leaving here and I'm glad of it. I've never been anywhere where they let the nurses talk back like they do here. In Alabama, the attending is the only one allowed to talk to the family and he does, so it's all coordinated. This group of nurses sides with the family and sets us up to be the bad guys."

"I don't leave often. If I go to the store, the nurses know when I'll be back. Don't they have some legal thing that requires my permission before they do things to her?"

"What you have to understand is we *have* talked to her. I heard Dr. Smith on the phone with her just the other night. He went over each of the possible outcomes. We can't help it if she forgets. Maybe she should call us to see what's going on. That might fit her schedule better. I'm sure whoever is on call could deal with her."

"Well, so the pulmonary guys said the lung was blown. *We* didn't know that. Why are *we* always blamed for not telling her? She didn't ask the right service."

"He said changing her trach wasn't considered a procedure. OK. So what should I call those things I don't want them doing to her without me here?"

"What she has to understand is . . ."

NADINE'S SECRET

Amy Haddad

The women in the adult intensive care unit for psychiatric patients slept down one hallway of the L-shaped unit, the men down the other. At the point where the two hallways converged, the night shift staff usually pulled a card table out of the day room so they could sit in the intersection and monitor both hallways. The first patients to arise in the morning were usually the smokers, who would walk down to the card table to get a light. Sometimes the patients would pull a chair out from the day room and sit in silence while they smoked their first cigarette of the day.

As head nurse of this unit, I was often there very early and very late. One particular morning I arrived early to meet with one of the night staff before she went home for the day. As I stood exchanging whispered small talk with the night staff, a door opened down the women's hallway. Nadine emerged from her room and slowly made her way down the hallway to us. Nadine was a middle-aged woman who had been diagnosed with manic-depressive psychosis. On admission, she was in a full-blown, flamboyant manic phase. She had run all of her credit cards to the limit, hadn't slept for days, and was picked up for disorderly conduct when she refused to leave a bar at closing time. When the police brought her to the emergency room, she was still dressed in a red sequined cocktail dress, singing at breakneck speed as loudly as she could. Now with medication she was subdued, at least in demeanor. However, she still wore the vestiges of her former outrageous self by applying makeup every morning as though she were going to appear on stage.

For a moment, it looked as if Nadine was naked as she walked towards us, but as she got closer I could see the faint outline of a flame-orange baby-doll nightgown. The nylon was so thin that it was essentially transparent except for ruffles around the low-cut neckline and arms. She wore gossamer orange panties that were no more than two triangles connected by string. As Nadine leaned forward with a cigarette hanging from her mouth, she said, "Got a light?" I was momentarily speechless as I lit her cigarette.

"Nadine," I began, "I'm afraid you won't be able to wear that nightgown around here."

"Why?"

"It's just not appropriate. You cannot wear it here. You'll have to wear something else that's not so sheer."

"*All* my nighties are like this. I like them bright, cool, and sexy."

"If all your nighties are like this, then you will have to wear a patient gown."

Nadine paused and smoked. She leaned against the door and seemed to be completely at ease, even though the two psychiatric technicians and I could see everything—her sagging, ample breasts, the pouch of her stomach over the top of the bikini pants, her pubic hair. Nadine rolled her eyes and sighed. She ran her fingers through her disheveled hair, which was dark at the roots and bright red on the ends from the dye she used during her manic phase.

"Those patient gowns are ugly. Come on. I'm not hurting anyone. Besides, my butt will hang out in the back," Nadine countered.

I was ready for this argument. "You can wear two patient gowns. Put one on the regular way and the other like a coat to cover your backside."

I heard some of the male patients rousing from sleep, so I followed my words with action. I did not want Nadine standing in the hallway dressed like that when the male patients came out. I opened the linen closet and got out two gowns. "Here," I said in my most professional voice. "Put out your cigarette and put these on in the bathroom."

"You know what?" Nadine said over her shoulder as she walked to the bathroom, "You're no fun."

The next morning, Nadine was again the first one up. I was pleased to see that she had on the requisite patient gowns, front and back. She pulled a chair out of the day room, sat down, and yawned loudly. A few minutes later, three male patients made their way down the hall to the communal bathroom. The noise of the toilets flushing and water running inevitably woke up the rest of the patients on the unit. As the women patients awoke and opened their doors, the scene down their hallway was like some badly colorized version of *Night of the Living Dead*. One by one every female patient shuffled down the hall in various stages of drug or sleep-induced stupor decked out in neon shades of green, red, purple, yellow, fuchsia, blue and orange, transparent baby-doll nighties and matching bikini pants. Although the nighties were of similar style and size, the women were not. Some of the women barely fit into the flimsy gowns, others swam in them, the bikini pants held up by a hand.

Some of the early risers on the men's side of the hall ran back to their rooms and pulled their roommates out of bed to come see the sight. Eventually, the staff and all of the male patients stood at the end of the hallway and dumbly watched this garish procession. Nadine smiled slightly and said, "Got a light?"

BACK TO SQUARE ONE
Barbara Jessing

First Recollections

I can remember first meeting her, though it was more than eight years ago, and though she was one of dozens that came and left again—a young mother with four children like stairsteps behind her, and a man's fedora angled over one eye. Living on AFDC was an uphill struggle to most, but she took it as a challenge. She knew they would make it. Things would be better. Their needs were few and simple.

She had come to the parent support group I led because she wasn't happy with her way of discipline. "I hit my kids too much. It's not working. I want to do it differently."

There was a shadowy man in the background—not the children's father, but living in, and a high-profile disciplinarian. I never met him, never asked to, and only spoke to him once by phone, after he was imprisoned.

Other parents in the group saw her spark, too; she emerged as a natural leader. She could think from a child's perspective as few others could. She realized that her kids were not just short and obstinate adults. She knew that they got into things because they were curious and driven to learn. She knew how to rechannel that curiosity in safer ways. The kids loved it and thrived on it.

One day, she told me they were leaving, she, the children, and her boyfriend. She had packed one plastic bag full of clothes for each of them and gotten rid of everything else they owned. They were leaving for a new life in a neighboring state. She asked me to help her find the name of an agency there so she could join a parent support group when she got settled. But getting settled never happened.

A Year Later

When I saw her again, a year or so later, I was shocked. She had aged far more than a year. Barely into her 20s when I'd last seen her, she now seemed to have edged up on middle age. Her face was haggard. She was heavier. She was deeply discouraged. She had called me to ask for some help to find food. When we arranged for delivery, I found that she and the children were living in a tent and a car at a city park outside of town.

They had been evicted from the apartment they'd been staying in and she was trying to save up enough money to get into another place. In the late October chill, this park was full of homeless families, laundry hung from rope lines around tents, and cars made into makeshift homes. Finally, the cold wore them down and a child with asthma became increasingly ill. Until they could afford a place, they all camped in one bedroom of another family's apartment.

That housing solution, and the next as well, turned out to be temporary. I heard from her again the next summer. "I've been evicted. I have no money, no car, and have nowhere to go."

My job had changed by this point. Most of what I did now took place by appointment, on the hour, and in the office. It was supposed to be less about casework and less about advocacy, and more about family therapy. I was supposed to be referring her to some other service. But I went out, anyway, bumping down an unpaved inner city alley and knowing where to stop because her daughter, now maybe nine or ten, marked the place, sitting on a ragged fence and sobbing in transparent and absolute sorrow. I have often wondered what it was about, and why I never asked about it.

She never expected me to do it for her. Her requests for help were reticent and specific and were aimed at "getting a grip on things," as she would often say over the years.

I remember, that time, learning a vivid lesson about triage: with all that was wrong for her, where did it make sense to begin—should the little bit of money she had go into a home, or a car, or food? We talked about it and she pieced it together— "first a car, because then I'll be able to drive around to find a job and a house. Meanwhile we can live in it if we have to." It would not have been my first choice, but it made sense to her. She breathed in deep relief once she had decided, and she was back on her feet.

Another Year
It was another year or more till I saw her again. She phoned to say something was terribly wrong and she needed to see me. She arrived with her eleven-year-old daughter, who had just revealed to her mother that she had been sexually abused by the man the mother had loved and trusted for many years.

I told her that I had to make a child abuse report and I could see in her face all the devastation that would result, but she did not resist, she agreed, and we talked to the police officers together. Blessedly, this was one of the times that the system works as it should. The child was interviewed by a trained, sensitive, female officer. The man was promptly arrested, and the case was investigated.

He eventually pleaded guilty and the child did not have to endure public testimony aimed at discrediting her experience.

But this woman was devastated. There was the betrayal to deal with. For all his faults this man had provided the structure that the family needed to operate. Without him, she was unable to maintain a routine, and over the next year there was a steady deterioration. She looked numbed out and seemed increasingly disorganized. Discipline was erratic, meals haphazard, housework and laundry far beyond the survival level at which they were struggling. She tried to work but could not afford child care. She was diagnosed with diabetes but could not afford health care. She would work until she was too sick, or until the children, usually left in the care of the eleven-year-old daughter, precipitated a crisis that demanded that she give up the job. Then she would stay home until dire financial necessity forced her out again. "I'm back to square one," she would often tell me.

There were crises with the kids. Their stability rested on hers, and when hers was lacking, they acted up. The cumulative effects of these years of uncertainty were wearing on them. Surviving was no longer the adventure it had been when they were small.

Bits and pieces of her history emerged as we talked through these rough times. I heard her oldest son tell her once, as we struggled with why he was having such trouble in school, "I can't sleep when you're drinking and yelling."

She told me that she had been born addicted to drugs that her mother had used during pregnancy. She was in fragile condition during the first few weeks of life, alone in a hospital while her mother suffered a breakdown. She told of a childhood marked by violence and alcoholism and living in the constant terror of being beaten. Though her father was her chief tormentor, she remained fiercely loyal and felt bound to care for him in his last illness. Her grief when he died was overwhelming. "I should have been there. I could have done something."

When I looked back, I could see the pattern over the years— she too had long been dependent on alcohol and marijuana to combat the stresses, the bleakness, the poverty, the discouragement. It was such a constant backdrop that she never spoke of it, and in those days I was still learning to ask those harder questions.

Meanwhile, her health deteriorated—she developed migraines in addition to diabetes. She was insulin-dependent and had great difficulty managing the medication, the stress level, and the diet that all contribute to treating this chronic condition. Twice in one year, she was hospitalized for several days of intensive care—an expensive consequence of not being able to afford regular insulin or health maintenance.

She eventually broke down under the burden. She turned on her daughter in a moment of rage and struck her. School officials, alarmed at the girl's appearance, reported child abuse. The children, found in a dirty, disorganized home and without adequate food or clean clothing, were placed in foster care, and their mother entered chemical dependency treatment. The Juvenile Court required, in addition to her treatment, that she find and maintain employment and housing.

My part in the plan was to see her for individual psychotherapy. The judge told her that she needed to do grief work over the death of her father and deal with the trauma in her own family history.

But she was also deprived of medical benefits, because a parent loses medical eligibility when children are removed from the family. She had no means to take care of her health.

Back to square one. She would find a fast-food, minimum-wage job, but would eventually lose it because of absences due to illness. She had no phone to call in if ill. In times that she was well enough to work, she also had to cope with unreliable transportation. It seemed like an endless struggle just to keep going. The prospect of getting it all together—making a home for four growing kids—seemed to get further away, not closer. In between jobs she would seek out health care, usually in an emergency, at the county's health care clinic for indigent adults. By the time she made it through the long bureaucratic process of determining eligibility, she was often working again, and would thus have to go further into debt for the crisis medical care she had already received, and she was no closer to being able to afford preventive or maintenance care. She would get close to the point of affording an apartment, and would find other obstacles in the way—a debt for utilities from some long-ago winter that would have to be paid off before she had a chance of renting again. Back to square one.

I remember the wintry day that she called from a phone booth not too far from the office, barely hanging on. I got somebody to take me out to find her and bring her back to the office. I remember the moment when I realized that the absurd choice before me was to do grief work or find insulin. After a frustrating morning on the phone trying to find some public or private source of help—a struggle she was in no shape at that moment to handle—I took her to a drug store and bought the insulin myself.

I was feeling a bit of shame. There's an emphasis in our field now on maintaining proper boundaries, with the implication that those who do not are overfunctioning, co-dependent and other compound words even more dreadful. Emotional disengagement was expected. Technically—though no one forbade it—it was not part of my job to go find people in phone booths or pay for their medicine. I was aware of stretching the limits of what I usually do.

I remember the day that she sat in my office in absolute despair, and as we talked I diagrammed the incredibly complex and interdependent spiral of problems. Which one was it that, if properly touched, would promise to be the keystone on which all the others balanced? I remembered what I had learned from her about triage—what seemed like the most important, first step.

I used to think that the keystone was money—I remember a daydream in which I would have the money to lend and invest for her, and others like her, so that with decent and stable housing as a foundation, healthy family life would flourish.

Then I watched her race through the spending of all of a modest legal settlement from a car accident, with no appreciable change in her quality of life—she didn't use it to get into an apartment, or to buy a reliable car. I don't know what happened to it.

When I asked her what she thought the root of her problem was, she always found fault with herself: "I am lazy. I have had too many bad habits for too many years." I never heard her rage at the injustices I could see—that in this rich country, she had no access to health care, could not find and keep adequate housing, could not afford quality child care; could not live decently on AFDC. She quietly absorbed the blame: "I'm lazy."

So how much had to do with her—her motivation, strength of character, faith, persistence—those inborn qualities that can be sheltered and nurtured as long as there is some life, but cannot regenerate once they die?

More than I realized. This is the part I had trouble seeing and understanding.

And how much had to do with the time, place, and situation she was born into—the triple disadvantages of gender, deprivation, and violence?

More than she realized. This was the part that she could not see as well as I could.

The Last Year

In the fall of that last year, she was hospitalized after a drinking binge of several days that sent the diabetes out of control. The diagnosis was malnutrition. Her grip on life was precarious.

The next time I saw her, she summed up that experience like this: "God kicked me in the butt." But she was hopeful. "Back to square one," which she said again this time, sounded more like a fresh start and less like a discouraging slide.

This was the day that it occurred to me that she was unlikely to be able to handle having all four of her troubled kids come home at the same time. So we talked about trying it step by step—focus on one child, rebuild that relationship, work out the adjustments, and then shift to the next.

I saw the old spark that day. She was excited. It seemed possible. She felt she could do it. I promised to help her call a meeting to present this idea to her probation officer and others working on the case. It was her daughter, she felt, who needed to come home first.

Five days before she died, we spoke on the phone about holiday plans for her children, and I helped her make some arrangements for gifts she wanted to give them. And she had rented an apartment, she told me excitedly—a place for her and her daughter to live. Her probation officer had been receptive to the idea of phasing the children back into their mother's home on a gradual schedule.

Monday morning—a message marked urgent, a probation officer's name. Before I call, I know it is about a death, but not whose.

The probation officer, with a rapid-fire delivery that skates over the pain, gives me the few details that are known at this point: she was found dead over Thanksgiving weekend. The manner of death had not been determined, but the scene suggested self-infliction.

A couple of days later, a message slip confirms it: the coroner rules that the cause of death was self-inflicted.

Her Mother

A few days before Christmas, I call on her mother, whom I had never met, to pay respects and to bring the gifts for the children that their mother had planned to give them. She is bewildered and disbelieving of what has happened to her daughter, and questions the coroner's verdict. She does not believe that her daughter would have killed herself now.

I am able to tell her about the fondness with which I heard her daughter talk about her. She had found a sense of support, of reconnection with her mother, at the end of her life that had been missing when her needs were more overwhelming. I recalled the day she had appeared for an appointment we had, with her hair done attractively, and with makeup on. "My Mom helped me do it. I think she's trying to lift my spirits."

That night, I dream of war-ravaged countries, and images of mothers nearly starving under conditions of extreme deprivation, yet continuing to sacrifice pieces of themselves, so that some piece of a child will still live. Hope stays alive for the next generation.

Closure

I needed some closure. I needed to find out from the other professionals who knew her what they thought happened—not just the death, but the frustrating life heading up to it. Could we have done better, or differently? Was there something we missed in those last few months, when it seemed things were finally improving?

As we sat down with coffee that winter morning, the probation officer flipped open a police report to somewhere near the middle, to a neatly drawn diagram. It was a stunning moment: I realized I was looking at a sanitized portrayal of a crime scene, with an anonymous gingerbread figure sprawled in the corner.

Geometric shapes had been precisely stenciled in and labeled to represent the layout of the apartment where she died.

I think about the tidy genograms I construct with families, the drawings with their tiered generations of squares, circles, boundaries, and hierarchies, and the function it serves for me of forcing order onto chaos.

Her Daughter

At fifteen years of age, her daughter looks strikingly like the young mother I had first met seven or so years ago.

She'd been willing to come see me, to talk with someone who had known her mother for a long time.

She was apologetic about the flapping sole of her sneaker: "I need shoes but my foster mother hasn't noticed."

"Is it hard for you to ask for what you need?" I ask.

There was a thoughtful pause. "No, not really. It's just that I wouldn't have needed to tell my mom. She just would have known. She would have noticed and taken care of it, even if we were short of money. My foster mom is used to kids who get in her face and yell about what they want."

Thus everyday, normal suburban family life, intended to be protective and healing of this child, becomes a constant irritant in her grief.

On the phone I had asked her foster mother about how this daughter was handling the loss of her mother. There had been very little outward reaction, she told me. Her grades dropped, she was quieter, she stayed in her room more.

Today this young woman tells me that for quite some time after her mother's death, she told none of her friends, no one knew at school. It left her with a daily life in which she could imagine, if sufficiently numbed, that this terrible loss had never happened. But recently, for a class project, she wrote and presented a speech about her mother. "Now," she tells me with a small smile, "everyone knows about her." She found a way to speak about her mother in the way she remembered her—for her courage, for the difficulty of her struggle, and not for the failure and weakness that others saw.

We spent a total of three hours together, some of it silently, some of it just listening, some of it sharing the memories each had, from different perspectives. She worried a lot about her mother's soul. Would she be judged as harshly in the afterlife as she was here on earth? She was sensitive and defensive toward those who saw her mother primarily for her flaws and weakness.

"I am sorry," she tells me one day, "that I ever told." She is referring to her disclosure of incest, and later, to telling about her mother's angry beating of her, which led to the removal of her and her siblings from the home.

"Things were bad, but what happened because I told was far worse."

In her mind, telling about her own mistreatment was something she was not entitled to do. It was the first domino to fall, and the direct result of it was the destruction of her family and eventually her mother's death. If only she'd been silent—the thought hangs.

I am stricken by the echoes of her mother in what she says, and I feel compelled to say so. I know that kids need to learn from their own experiences, and that adult words of warning are weak by comparison—but this is one lesson I hope she can learn without suffering as much as her mother did.

"Your mother did this too, she blamed herself for everything, even things she could have no control over. She blamed herself for far more than she could do anything about. It overwhelmed her, and she couldn't even deal with some of the stuff that was her responsibility, that she could do something about. I hope you don't make the same mistake."

Shortly thereafter, I received word that the children would be moving to a neighboring county to live with their mother's sister, and we did not meet again.

In Retrospect

I still think of her often. I am sorry for the moments of pain and despair in which her life ended—though what and how and why it happened may never be known. But what I learned from her shapes the work I have done with every other family since.

I think of how much she was in tune with her children when

they were very young, How she loved and played with them and knew their ways of thinking and feeling. No matter how many parents' education curricula I write, this is really the only point I ever want to make.

She comes to mind when I search for a family's strengths—the spark that can start the healing. It is almost always there. When I can't find it, I know now to let go. That this is a hurt I cannot help to heal.

I think of her in my effort to ask the hard questions in the right way, to maintain a perspective in which I can see those questions emerge from the background, without losing focus on the person they are about.

And almost every day, I am treading a fine line with someone, seeking out the right balance between blame and responsibility, and whenever I do this, I think of her.

I think of her in my greater urgency to work with intensity, to turn up the heat under a low-key style when I need to. What if I had gathered together the energy, the years of low-level influence I had with her, into a single brilliantly timed and life-changing burst?

I worked with her as if we had forever, and we didn't.

But there is something to be said for the longer, slower pace as well. I had a glimpse of three generations in this family's life, and I know that in families some changes come slow as glaciers. If you are in too big a hurry to be done with it, you could be long gone before the results take hold.

OAT CELL

Audrey Shafer

Huge arms like bellies of dead fish
    kinked veins and shriveled legs—
The victim did not answer questions, did not say
One word
    only lay, cyanotic and breathing oxygen.

I wanted to leave.

But we manipulated her into a sitting position,
    left impressions of our fingers on her arms,
    listened at her ribbed back between
Old age spots on the rotting peel.

As we lowered her, strands of her long wiry hair
    and the small weight of a fibrotic breast
Brushed my arm.

We palpated the subcutaneous metastasis
    —Rub the skin to determine the adhesions.
The granite edges nauseated me.

I do not know how much pain she felt
    as she stared and lay—
And breathed from the green metal tank.

INTENSIVE CARE WAITING ROOM

Judy Hopkins Schaefer

The gray vapor of death
Reaches into the enclave
Like infinite snake or fog
Mocking teasing striking
Moving always moving
Turning flipping running
Striking
Slithering around ankles
Passing touching soft tissue of faces
A caress
Offering a terminal final promise
Loving coaxing fluttering
In a stagnant cave
Stones blocking exit or entry
Striking
And on another floor in another room
A baby cries with a first surprise
First gasp of father's air
And on another floor in another room
A young man flirts
And walks on a virgin wooden leg
He winks and calls the leg Margaret
And on another floor in another room
A sallow nurse
Pulls tight the sterile
Sheets on a freshly made bed
Like ice across a white pond
And a maid down a tunnel

Moves thin shoulders hips hands
Mops a blood-stained floor
According to aseptic technique
Striking
They huddle and wait
And they wait
According to the gray rules of death

(first appeared in *Wild Onions II* [Pennsylvania State University College of Medicine, 1987])

WHEN TOO MUCH IS ENOUGH ALREADY!

Kate Brown

Health care crisis
in prices keeps rising.

"How much is enough to pay?"

My salary's paid from
the profits of suffering.

"How much makes your efforts worthwhile?"

You can't pay me enough.

"But enough is enough!"

Who are you to say so, and why?

"I'm a child without a future."
"I'm someone without the same."
"Me, I'm a father, a farmer
without any fields;
my baby there took them away."
"I can't see to buy glasses."
"There's no money for medicine
so each night passes slowly,
waiting without knowing why."

Then raise barriers to access!
Raise all of your taxes!
Who would deny we care for your pains?

But don't stop this engine,
or you'll be buried by morning.
Our sights are on plenty,
and enough is too little:
lay-ins with inlaid wood
in the halls, monitors and bells,
shiny newest of everything,
soft lighting, soft slippers,
beds to float pain from the night.

Your life,
my livelihood,
depend on this way.
And whose life isn't worth
a monkey's liver nowadays?

THE WAITING ROOM

Susan Ogborn

Everyone is sucking their thumbs.
Babies, children, children with children,
Everyone is sucking their thumbs.
It hits me harder than the smell of vomit,
Or the vacant stares of the junkies.
In this plot of urban landscaping we call an emergency room,
Everyone is sucking their thumbs.

KEEPING PERSPECTIVE

Susan Ogborn

Two women, two stories.

She smiled and said, "I'm in real trouble, aren't I?" when I walked in.

My stomach hurt too much to do anything besides nod. So I went clinical and said the appropriate words: "It has nothing to do with your performance."

"We have decided to decentralize your functions . . . ," and I realized, with horror, that I had become an administrator after all. She burst into red, blotchy, embarrassing tears, and I cursed these cheap, scratchy Kleenex we keep around here.

We tried to find her husband and settled for the physical relief provided by driving her home. Her cries sounded like my dog when she's trying to get up from sleep: "Where am I going to go? What am I doing to do?"

And then she said "thank you" as I left.

KEEPING PERSPECTIVE — REPRISE

Susan Ogborn

"You know," she said, "this just isn't working out."

I thought I'd just come in to confirm a meeting.

"You know, you never have been able to do for us what we needed to have done. Costs are such a concern right now, and so I think it's time for us to sever this relationship."

All the faces, all the tears, all the fears of others I'd shared as a voyeur, flashed before me. And I smiled. Grateful for the freedom.

Dying is far worse than death.

Vulnerability
and
Voice

UNTITLED

Jolene Siemsen

She came into the room smiling.
"This is the real thing," said the interpreter.
"Sientese," I said, gesturing to the chair, grateful
    for my limited Spanish.
I asked her questions about cancer and illness.
"Only Americans talk of dying of cancer," she
    said.
I asked her questions about cancer and illness.
"Look in the eyes, you can tell by the eyes," she said.
I looked in her eyes.
I asked her questions about cancer and illness.
"The *curanderas* use objects and herbs for
    healing.
They have their own way of speaking.
No one else understands them."
She looked at me.
"That's all," she said. She stood.
that's all that's all that's all
whispered ancestor spirits.
holders of ancient wisdom
written in Aztec
kept in jars and pots
herbs animals
stones
goat's milk
"That's all," she said.
She smiled.
She left the room.

(first published in *Nightingale Songs* [November 1993])

POTTED MOUSE SANDWICH

Veneta Masson

Sweetheart! Nurse!
What are you doing?
Why have you got
your head in that bag?

> *I'm throwing out the wet*
> *newspapers and the dried-up*
> *food that fell on the floor.*

Well, that's what comes
of having a delicatessen
here on the bed.
It can't be helped.
Now go to the icebox
find that can of potted meat
and make me a sandwich
would you, Sweetheart?

> *Ms. Jackson, I'm here to fix*
> *your leg not your dinner.*
> *Nurses today can't cater*
> *as much as they used to.*

Not later, now—
the potted meat
and two slices of bread
and that hallway light
needs a bulb put in.
It's much too dark in there.

Nurse, where are you?
Where did you go?

I'm stuck in the hall.
I stepped into something.

The potted meat
and a little French dressing!

There's a long tail
sticking out from the side
of my shoe

Stale? It's not stale.
It's only been in there a week.
Step on it, Sweetheart.
I haven't eaten all day.

I stepped on it, yes
and now my shoe is stuck
in a gooey mousetrap
along with a gooey mouse.
Can you hear me, Ms. Jackson?
I'm caught!

That's right, the potted
meat is what I want
and sprinkle it with
sugar, if you please.

ASKING FOR DIRECTION
Amy Haddad

He fell dead in the parking lot of a convenient mart.

His wife never learned to drive,
had never written a check,
never made a move without asking him first.

And now they ask,
"What would you like us to do?"
"How aggressive should we be?"

And she tells them she must leave because
her neighbor is giving her a ride and it's her only way home.

When she visits again, they say,
"We suspect permanent brain damage.
Shall we resuscitate him if his heart stops beating?"

Day after day,
"Shall we discontinue the ventilator?"
"Shall we continue artificial nutrition and hydration?"
Waiting, she holds his limp hand,
silently begs him to tell her what to do.

Since he doesn't answer,
she slips out to catch a ride with her neighbor.

THE PILOT

Amy Haddad

He has worn the same clothes for three days,
still has on his trenchcoat, hasn't bothered
to take it off, hasn't shaved either.
He absently bends down the edges of
a Styrofoam coffee cup, as fatigue
circles his eyes. He says, "I've been a pilot
for years. I know what it means to handle
stress, to be responsible for life
and death decisions. I feel like I've been
flying for days, watching those monitors,
trying to read them for signs of where
to turn." He raises his hands as if
clutching the yoke of a plane. "I feel
like I've been at the controls for days
with no break." His mother lies moribund
in the ICU, heart beating, breathing
but gone. A neighbor ran to a pay
phone to call 911, and no one
knows how long she was dead before they
revived her. "I tried to get here as
fast as I could. I haven't seen her
in six months. Why the hurry to decide?
Do they need the bed? I just need some
time. She's my mom. If I could just land
for a while. You know, rest a bit.
Then I could say good-bye."

THE EAR

Kate Brown

I always imagined comas were quiet states of being, or at least muffled. The body's immobility implied an inner stillness and an impenetrable absence of feeling. No pain, no consciousness, a floating existence beyond the touch of human connection.

But I was wrong. I can hear everything acutely in painful, unending detail. I have no way to dampen the incoming sounds, to change the channel, to alter or even modulate the constant bombardment of audial sensations now comprising the tedium of my days. Even the most minute sounds that would otherwise be subsumed into the background now demand my unceasing attention. I hear the gurgle of the fluid dripping through a tube into my arm, the silent flip of the clock hands in their relentless journey round the diameter of time, the constant, piercing high-pitched beeping of the machines monitoring my stasis. Harnessed to a ventilator, my breaths whisper and whoosh in and out, steady and predictable as a metronome. Always and underneath everything else is the persistent pulse of my heart muscle. I yearn to stop the beating, to break the eternal monotony.

I am an ear, and nothing more. A receptacle for sound, a bottomless pit that is always full, never overflowing. A black hole, passively engulfing every decibel of noise.

And I have no way of letting anyone know. Occasionally they test me, clapping in my ear. What, to see if I flinch? I hate it. Friends come and cry and talk to me. I can't feel their touch, but I can hear their hands on my forehead. I hear their gentleness, their pain, and their fear. And I hate how much I need their love. Hell within hell is when the night nurse leaves on the TV to "keep me company." How could such caring be so misplaced?

Some think I can't hear because I can't register a response. Others think I can hear in ways that are beyond hearing. I can hear, but that's all I can do. That's the point. I have tried everything to respond. I ache from emanating sincerity, intimacy, even rageful screaming, but all my efforts stay hidden within me, resonating like echoes of the sea in a conch shell buried beneath the sand.

I remember assembling a plastic model of an ear when I was a child. It was a beautiful structure when completed, and I kept it on my desk for years, marveling at its labyrinthine depth and my own cleverness. Careful sequential directions guided my efforts to first paint, then glue the many intricate plastic pieces. The names of the parts were magical: the stirrup, the tympanum, the cochlea, are all that remain with me today. I remember having to ask my father to help me with a particularly tricky set of glued connections. Up until then the directions had been clear, but they fell into vagueness at this point. Ambiguity should have been expected, for we had reached the "inner ear," the most vulnerable sanctum, the place of deepest mysteries where hearing takes place.

Now I understand that the mystery is not in hearing. Anyone with the equipment can hear, it is merely a sensory response to stimulation. No, the divine purpose of the ear is not for hearing, but for listening. Though not mentioned in my directions for the model ear, listening is the ear's true power. A listening ear can tune out noise, make meaning of sounds. But a listening ear depends on the body's mobility to move it in and out of range, and on the selective depth and vision provided by the eyes. The listening ear can function only as a player with all the other senses in concert orchestrated by the mind. Together, this swirling dance of perceptions turns otherwise random sounds into information, music, love, food for the soul. By itself, the ear is unfulfilled, a mockery of human capacities.

Silenced in the static din of my current existence, I remember my grandmother's moral exclamations when she was reading the newspaper. Some new invention, some exploit by the outrageous, some atrocity of human invention, would trigger her astonishment. Out loud to no one in particular she'd announce, "Well, now I've heard everything!"

LAST RIGHTS

Tess Yelland/marino

Tight-faced, they found and cornered her at work.
As quick as hammers pounding down a wall
the words came hard and nailed that little quirk
of honesty so fast she held the rail.

"Who were you to say he was a dying
man, though he lay white, his life thread thin?
How were you to know the speed his flying
heart would race away from bone and skin?

He was hopeless, yes, beneath that tent
of filmy gauze, but who were you to say
his fate was hinged on prayer—our magic spent?
Who knows, he might have lived another day."

"He held my hands and asked the truth," she said.
Then turned away to smooth the empty bed.

(first published in *Nightingale Songs* [January 1993])

BILLY

Claudia Peyton

I remember my first day on the job at the state hospital. The charge nurse described the patients I would be working with as having such a low mentality that they wouldn't be able to recognize that they were drowning if submerged in a swimming pool. Essentially, they were completely unaware of the world and themselves.

We went on a tour of the ward. It was a dark place with a high wax shine on the floor. The sun shone through windows set close to the ceiling and cast long rays of light with dust falling through it. On the floor at the ends of those rays were several men, sitting and squinting at us as we walked by. The charge nurse showed no recognition of them, only an ongoing monologue of what tasks I would be expected to complete during the evening shift.

The staff were eager to see a new face, as now the rungs on the ladder could shift up. I was the person to take charge of the lowest-functioning group, those patients with the least ability. Those that were incontinent and unaware of it, those who grabbed food from others' trays when in the chow hall and who stuffed two and three slices of bread into their mouths and then choked. My group was known to the staff as the grabbers and stuffers, the worst of the mentally retarded. The members of this group were introduced to me as they sat in a large room on hard yellow plastic couches which outlined its perimeter. Most were middle-aged men who were autistic in their behaviors, sitting, pacing, or reclining on the tile floor. They did not acknowledge me but stared blankly or flipped mop strings or regurgitated food into their hand to re-examine it. Some had urinated in their pants and soaked their tennis shoes in the process, leaving small puddles on the floor.

I felt sick—nauseated and overwhelmed; the smell of urine and feces permeated the air. The patients had food in their hair and food mixed with drool on their shirts. These fourteen men were my responsibility to care for, to feed and to bathe in the eight hours ahead.

No amount of education could have prepared me for this. At first I wanted to run in the other direction or to at least maintain my professional, objective demeanor, to distance my inner self from this gut-wrenching picture. Yet, I found in our many hours together how each did have a feeling person inside. Over the months I found that nurturing care had not been a part of this group's history. They were docile and fearful and, I thought, seldom communicated their needs or were heard if they did. Some were old, like Billy.

So many times I wondered how many people had been Billy's caregivers. He had been in the state hospital system since he was four—sixty years. Sixty years of different people to adjust to, sixty years of institutional life. Sixty years of being herded into a community shower room, disrobed together and hosed clean. Sixty years of wearing clothes that didn't fit and being told to go sit down.

After months of working with Billy as if he were non-speaking, I tucked him in one night, and he whispered, "Hey lady, how's Percy?" What an overwhelming feeling. I wanted to burst into tears, to hug Billy and tell him how sorry I was that I didn't know where to find Percy. I said, for lack of another thought, "He's fine, Billy." Each night that week Billy asked me the same question until I asked Billy where I could visit Percy. He told me that he and Percy used to work "up to the morgue house together" and that Percy had given him a sailor hat. Then from under his arm and beneath his pajamas he pulled out a Navy knit cap, quickly showed it to me and then put it back under his arm.

I will never know who Percy was to Billy. Patients in the state hospital system had stopped working in the '60s, some fifteen years before. Yet, I know that Percy was ever-present to Billy and was someone that Billy had loved and lost.

RITUAL

Amy Haddad

She paces round the quiet room,
unable to stop. Right hand,
index finger only touching
every third brick vertically,
every twelfth brick horizontally,
avoiding the cracks in the floor,
softly repeating a personal
prayer that lasts as long as the trip
around the room.
Each trip takes her past the window;
she touches it in the center
each time, her right hand flat against
the locked metal screen. As she touches
the screen, she turns her head away as if
to avoid falling into the sky.
She does not stop to eat, carries
her food in her left hand; alone
or observed she continues her course.
Her family, not knowing what to do,
brings presents for her sixteenth birthday.
The boxes are brought to her, bedecked
in yellow flowers with violet
ribbons, pink stripes with a shiny blue
bow, scarlet kisses on white paper
stacked on the floor. Her pacing does
not stop, she gives the presents a
wide berth, leans over the packages,
right hand, index finger only
touching every third brick vertically,
every twelfth brick horizontally,
avoiding the cracks in the floor,
chanting a little louder as she does.

WASHING CORA'S HAIR
Amy Haddad

The first week of our community health nursing class, the instructors briefed us on the contents of our "black bags," how to wash our hands without water and soap, and the basic differences between taking care of patients in a hospital and in their homes. The second week of class, we were each given an abbreviated "case load" of three families. We would be responsible for all of the nursing care these families would need for fifteen weeks—the last semester of our nursing program. We were given reports from the community health nurses who had previously been in charge of our cases.

My friend Kathi had been assigned an elderly woman, Cora, who had suffered a cerebral vascular accident, or stroke. Cora was unable to move her left arm and leg as a result of the stroke. She also had motor aphasia—that is, she was unable to utter understandable sounds. Cora had not spoken for years.

The nurse told Kathi that she should take one of her classmates with her after the initial get-acquainted visit because it would take two of us to care for Cora. Kathi asked me to help her.

We drove to the older, southeast section of the city. I had been there many times as a little girl because my father grew up there. He would take us to dinner at an old restaurant in the neighborhood that served dumplings that looked like sponges and exotic meats like capon and sweetbreads. After dinner, as we walked to the car, he would point out the print store that used to be a movie theater and the building where he grew up over a garage that now bore the sign "Hempel Steel."

Kathi and I were not going to this familiar part of the old neighborhood, but down almost under a viaduct where the trucks from the stockyards roared by. The house we were to visit was small, white, and badly in need of a new roof and paint. It looked exactly like the house children draw, with the front door in the middle, a window on either side, and perhaps a dormer, but certainly no second story. The yard was overgrown, although you could see where a flower garden once bordered the length of the house. A few climber roses poked their heads bravely above the weeds and tall grass. A single aluminum kitchen chair with a cracked maroon vinyl seat stood forlornly on the front porch.

We waited on the porch for Cora's husband to answer the door. The tieback curtains at the front windows parted to reveal stacks of old magazines, newspapers, boxes, and other clutter, which made it impossible to see into the house. An elderly man opened the door a few inches, saw who was standing there, nodded briefly and held out the screen door to us. When we were inside, he slowly walked to a coat rack and put on a denim jacket and a bill cap. Still without speaking he went over to a bed along the wall, bent down, and kissed the bed's occupant. He nodded to us once more as he passed out the front door.

As he was saying his good-bye, my eyes became accustomed to the dark and I looked around the room. It appeared that we were standing in the living room. From the living room you could look straight back to the opposite end of the house to another door, which looked like it opened to an enclosed porch or pantry. There was just enough space for Kathi and me to stand side by side in a path cleared down the middle of the room. It was very dark because all the light from outside was blocked out. It was as if the belongings of a much larger house were all stuffed into this smaller house. Or perhaps the occupants had never thrown anything away for the last fifty years. Back issues of *National Geographic* and the *Saturday Evening Post* lined one wall. Baskets of folded clothes were piled one on top of the other next to the magazines. A bookshelf was loaded with photographs, a vase of plastic flowers, at least a dozen statues of horses from metal to ceramic, in addition to countless paperbacks shoved two deep on each shelf. Brown grocery sacks with unknown contents lined another wall. Boxes of Christmas decorations were precariously balanced on an old television set. Along the wall next to the kitchen were canned goods, dishes, plastic marga-rine tubs, and empty milk cartons piled almost to the ceiling.

I whispered to Kathi, "Have you ever seen this much junk?"

"I know what you mean. When I first came, I was afraid to move or touch anything for fear it would all come tumbling down on me," she whispered in response.

The house wasn't dirty, exactly, just crammed full, dark, and musty. Kathi and I were the picture of incongruity standing there like a white island with our students' uniforms, hose, and shoes. An efficiency kitchen with a miniature stove, refrigerator, and sink ran along one wall about midway through the room.

Kathi said, "I'll introduce you to Cora." Across from the kitchen counter, Cora lay in a twin bed that had been wedged into its space between boxes and sacks. Kathi and I had both adopted the senseless habit of talking loudly to patients who were unable to speak, so as Kathi introduced me, I shouted my hello. Our loud voices triggered ferocious barking, growling, and scratching from behind the back door. The door actually shuddered and shook as the dogs lunged against it.

Kathi said, "I forgot about those dogs."

I grabbed Kathi's arm and backed up. "How many are there? Can they get out?"

"I'm not sure how many or even what kind. Cora's husband just told me to leave the door shut and they wouldn't bother me. They kept that up the whole time I was here last week."

I could hear the dogs snuffling at the base of the door. I imag-ined that they were drooling as well.

Kathi ignored the din and said to me, "We're going to wash Cora's hair." She then repeated this to Cora, as if she hadn't heard what Kathi just said.

"We're going to wash your hair, okay?"

Cora just watched us from the bed. Her eyes followed our every move, but her face remained fixed and bland. She had two thick braids that ran along the length of her body, almost reach-ing her feet. Her hair was black, peppered with gray. Now I un-derstood why it would take two of us to wash Cora's hair.

Both Kathi and I had long hair down to the center of our backs. Since we were in our professional roles, we had both pulled back our hair and pinned it up so we could work without it falling into our eyes. Our hair seemed short compared to Cora's.

I asked, "How do you want to do this? Have you done it before?"

"No. The nurse said it takes two people though because Cora's pretty stiff."

Cora's long confinement in bed had made it impossible to position her in a chair and lean her head back. We decided, since we could not think of any alternative, that we would have to wash her hair with her in the bed. Washing the hair of a bedfast patient was one of the skills we had mastered in the first year of our nursing program. It is no small trick to not get the patient and the whole bed wet. In the hospital, we had the advantage of a "hair board," a nifty device that cradles the patient's neck and lets the water run down a trough off the bed to a wastebasket.

Of course we did not have a hair board, nor was Cora in a hospital bed. In fact, the bed Cora was in was quite low to the floor, which required a considerable amount of stooping to reach her. Preparations for washing Cora's hair were intense. We tried to verbally walk through the whole process, and as we did, we would hunt for the supplies we thought we would need. We found shampoo and old hair conditioner in a closet next to the bathroom. Of course, we reasoned, Cora needed conditioner on her hair, we used conditioner on our hair. We didn't appreciate at this point that conditioner would necessitate another rinse. To protect the floor from anticipated spills, we spread newspapers all around the head of the bed. I found a pitcher to pour the rinse water and a bucket to catch it. Kathi found lots of towels. We took the oilcloth off the kitchen table and put it under Cora to protect the mattress. We were ready to begin.

We got on either side of the bed and pulled the bed away from the wall on an angle so the head would be nearer the sink. We moved Cora so she lay diagonally on the bed, with her head hanging over the edge.

"This isn't going to work," Kathi said. "She can't hold her head up, and we can't let her head hang down like that. It looks uncomfortable."

Cora watched us from an upside-down perspective as we discussed what to do.

"I'll hold her head in my lap while you wash her hair," I responded.

I squatted down and cradled Cora's head in my lap. Our faces were quite close. I remember thinking how smooth and unlined her face was for someone her age. Her eyes were such a dark brown that you could hardly see the pupils. She stared up at me with wide, frightened eyes.

"Don't worry," I said. "We'll try not to get water in your eyes." She still looked frightened. Her left arm had fallen off the bed and dangled on the floor. I saw that she was clutching the other side of the mattress with her right hand.

"Kathi, this isn't working. Get her arm off the floor and let's move her further onto the bed," I said.

"It's okay, Cora," I told her as we rearranged her. "We won't let you fall."

I knelt on the newspapers this time because I didn't think I could squat the whole time. I supported Cora's head with my right hand.

Kathi unbraided her hair. This took a long time. When Cora's hair was undone it lay all over my lap, spilling onto the floor in a thick pile.

"This bucket isn't big enough to catch the water," Kathi noted. "I'll have to find something else." Kathi searched under the sink and disappeared into the bedroom for a while. She came back with the top of an old manual washer, a large galvanized tub. My grandmother had one in her basement that she used to wash delicates by hand.

"Where did you find that?" I asked.

"Never mind. You wouldn't believe it anyway."

Kathi arranged the tub under Cora's head and put all of her

hair in it. Kathi then poured pitcher after pitcher of water on Cora's hair. Then she began to shampoo. I helped with my free hand and tried to keep water and soap from Cora's eyes.

"We'll have to dump this water before we can rinse her hair or we'll never be able to lift it to the sink," Kathi said.

We moved Cora's head back on the bed and both tried to lift the washtub. Her wet, soapy hair hung in dark rivulets over the side of the bed and down on the floor. The washtub was far too heavy for us to lift. We only got it an inch or two off the floor before we had to set it down with a bang and a resulting splash. This noise set off the dogs again.

Kathi used the pitcher and I used a tin coffee pot to bail water out of the washtub until it was light enough to lift to the sink and empty. Then we repositioned Cora and rinsed her hair. We learned from our previous mistake and only rinsed to the point where we could empty the washtub. It took three rinse cycles to get all of the shampoo out of Cora's hair.

By the second shampoo we were both wet with sweat and water from the endless rinses. Every time Kathi rinsed Cora's hair, the water ran into my lap, through my uniform, underwear, pantyhose and into my shoes. My knees were black with newsprint from the wet papers. Our hair had come undone with the effort and was hanging limply in disarray around our faces. My arms were tired from holding Cora's head and Kathi was exhausted from hauling so much water back and forth. We did not do as good a job of rinsing the conditioner from Cora's hair as we should have, but our enthusiasm was flagging.

We moved Cora back on the bed. We noticed that Cora and the bed were soaked. We dried Cora off and changed the bed.

"How do you dry her hair?" I asked.

"We don't. We'll just comb it and braid it again. It dries on its own."

We towel dried Cora's hair as best we could then began the arduous task of combing out the tangles we had created. Kathi could only find one comb, so I took mine from my purse. The only way to comb Cora's hair without pulling too much was to start down at the ends and work our way up to her scalp. This job was even worse than washing her hair. Our progress was literally measured in inches.

Finally, we were able to run a comb down both sides without encountering any resistance. We approximated a center part and carefully and slowly braided each side, catching our breath, winding down. I began to straighten up the floor and put back the supplies and equipment we had used. Kathi pulled the covers up to Cora's chest and folded them neatly. Cora used her good arm to pull her limp left arm out from under the covers and laid it along her side. She reached up and arranged each braid as well.

"Well, we're all finished," Kathi sighed. "I'll go tell your husband."

I hadn't realized that Cora's husband had been sitting outside on that maroon kitchen chair the whole time we had been there. He had been sitting outside for more than two hours. I don't know if he sat there because this was his only time to be alone, or if he didn't have anywhere to go, or if he wanted to be close but felt that this was somehow a private ceremony at which men were not allowed. It was a brisk, early spring day that left his cheeks red and eyes teary. He removed his hat and hung up his denim coat.

"Thank you, girls," he said as he walked toward the bed.

He gently touched Cora's face and one braid as he said, "Hello, beautiful." Then he kissed her on the forehead. He shyly looked up at us and said, "She's always had such pretty hair. It's her crowning glory." We said good-bye and left, shivering on the way to the car in our wet clothes.

Kathi washed Cora's hair every week throughout the semester. Since it took so much time, Kathi had to convince a new friend to go almost every time. Some of us went more than once. Although the procedure became more streamlined, you could count on being there for at least an hour and a half.

At a care conference near the end of the semester, all of the students reported on their case load. Kathi summarized her visits to Cora and ended her comments by stating, "It's getting harder and harder to justify the visits to Cora. Her husband can take care of most of her needs. He just can't manage keeping her hair clean. Someone said we should just cut it off so it would be easier to keep clean."

My hand involuntarily went to the back of my neck and fingered my hair, which was bound into a ponytail. "Cut off her hair," I thought. "No one would cut off *my* hair if I didn't want them to." But I wasn't old, small, bed bound, and mute, my only protection an equally old and frail sentinel, keeping guard in a maroon vinyl chair on the front porch.

THE MOTHER
— THE PHYSICIAN

Lynne Willett

I walk into the room and marvel at the quiet.
No red lights and alarms, no IV pumps,
no bustle of my colleagues.
The fancy gizmos and techno-wizardry are gone now.
Only the quiet noise of the respirator remains.
The shades are drawn and the dimmed lights show
only the beautiful baby.

The medical marvels haven't worked.
After days of frenzy,
We admit this little girl is going to die.
Every medical thing has been done.
I can finally turn off the doctor in me.
Your own mother could not be here, beautiful child.
I will try my best to fill her shoes.
I allow the other-me to do the things the doctor-me cannot.
In the quiet, I hold you close in my arms,
Inspect your bruised body, kiss the places you might hurt.
I whisper "Your mommy and daddy love you."
I tell you that you won't be alone. I'll hold you
until the pain is gone, my tears falling on your cheeks.

I feel my own child move in my belly.
Trying to comfort us both?
Trying to say it will be all right?
I hold two children close and wonder
at life being given and life taken away,
that children should suffer. Who decides this, anyway?
I take pictures of you for your parents so they can always see

how beautiful you are.
I take one for me, so I will never forget.
Then I hold you close to me.
I hold you close.

CAN A GIGGLE BE LOVE?

Sister Cashel Weiler

When I came to your
department for my EEG,
it wasn't actually humorous,
my shaved head chuck full
of tumors, but I tried
to make jokes because,
well, . . . because,
you and I are the same age.

Don't see it as acceptance,
it makes me furious.
But laughter takes the
bite out of my loss,
and out of your realization
of our mortality, and
well, I didn't want you
to feel uncomfortable or
anything, because . . .
the tumors in my brain are
the kind you die from,
and you and I, well,
we're the same age.

It lightens my heart
to hear you bubbling
with laughter, because
though I try to hide it,
inside, well . . . my
courage rides with terror!

THE STORY OF DAVID
Ruth Purtilo

The last time I saw David, he was being wheeled by an ambulance attendant out the front doors of the rehabilitation center into the light springtime morning. But that was a long time ago, as we usually think of time.

OCTOBER 15

It was Monday morning and I was wishing the weekend were a day longer. Winters were too long up there on the Canadian border, the other seasons too short. Autumn is intense, a brilliant harbinger of the icy months ahead. It had been a full year of seasons since I had graduated as a physical therapist, and the cadence of the school year was beginning to give way to the new energies of a professional life.

Ken, the chief therapist, raised his voice. "Did you hear me, Ruth? I'm giving you a new patient. David. Dove into three feet of water and broke his neck at a party after running the winning touchdown at his homecoming game last week. 18 years old. 220 pounds. Big hunk of a guy. Lesion at C 4-5 . . . may not be complete. Too early to tell."

I knew the day had begun . . . but as with many days, I had no idea of the journey down which the first step of this day would lead me in the months ahead . . .

I looked at my new patient. "This is terrible," I thought to myself as I took in his large frame. "Poor guy."

My mind began to race.

"I wonder what I would do?"

"Wouldn't it be incredible if he would walk out of here?"

"He has no idea of what is ahead . . . probably a good thing."

I maneuvered the treatment table awkwardly, hitting the corridor walls as I went, until we were alone behind a curtain in the treatment booth. He glowered up at me. After the usual introductions and explanation that I'd be evaluating him, I said that we would start by seeing if he could wiggle his toes.

"Why are you asking me if I can wiggle my toes?" His voice was a snarl. "You know damn well I can't wiggle my toes. I can't wiggle anything, Tootsie, unless you wiggle them for me. I'm like one of those Kewpie dolls, waiting for you to make me wiggle."

I looked at him quizzically, amused momentarily by the differences in our images of him. He looked less like a Kewpie doll than a Goliath prepared to bring down the old David he was a few weeks ago. But I was irritated, too. "My name is Ruth," I said in my most professional monotone. "Don't call me Tootsie, please. We'll be working together for a long time. Try to wiggle. This foot."

The toes wiggled, ever so slightly.

"I have news for you. You can wiggle your toes. See? I know you can't see. It's because of that head gear they have you in. Take my word for it. There is some wiggling in your left foot up to the level of the metatarsals and a little lateral movement, even if you can't tell you're doing it."

He was taken aback for a moment, but only a moment.

"I can wiggle my toes. Big fucking deal. What are you going to do with me, Tootsie Ruth? Why don't you do what they did in Rome? You don't know what they did in Rome? I'll tell you what they did. They threw guys like me to the lions."

"I have no intention of throwing you to the lions."

NOVEMBER 15

We worked together, more or less together, for four weeks. He stopped calling me Tootsie and I let my voice modulate a little. We liked each other, given the circumstances. Unfortunately, there was very little further evidence that he was going to gain much more motor function. But then, it was early, and in this arena time is the hedge against That Moment of Reckoning. As Ken said, "It's too early to tell."

Following the rehabilitation conference that week I announced the rehab team's decision enthusiastically: "We're going to stand you up in the parallel bars."

He stared in disbelief. He sounded incredulous when he began his response to this unexpected turn of events. "You must be kidding! You couldn't hold me up. I'm 220 pounds. I have no strength in my hands, no muscles in my trunk or legs." A pause. Then, explosively, "Why the hell are you going to stand me up?"

I explained, in the voice trained to confer my authority, "We think it will help your bones, also work any muscles that might be trying to kick in in your lower extremities."

He asked no more questions and I pushed his chair towards the bars, an orderly walking on either side. We positioned the chair at the end of the bars.

"OK!" I ordered, facing him and bending over to pull him up out of the sitting position, "Push him from behind! Push! His hips snapped forward as I pulled them to me and flung my arms tight around his trunk to hold it upright. My kneecaps crashed against his. "OK. OK. I've got his knees locked. Here! Tie his hands to the bars. Wait. Wait. Stop!! No. There! OK. I've got him. OK. Keep the chair there just in case." I was breathing heavily. "You OK, David? OK? Good!!" We stood locked in a tight embrace of dancers or clowns. But there was no dance floor and no circus tent. I felt close to him. I was close to him. I disappeared deep into my professional voice when I asked: "You're not light-headed are you? Good! How does it feel?"

DECEMBER 10

It was cold in the bedroom. The alarm went off and I drew myself more deeply under the down comforter. My first thoughts were about not wanting to go to work. It was a way of thinking about David. He'd lost a lot of weight. Down to 180 now. Forty pounds gone from the linebacker. Oh, well. That was to be expected. Better for him. I knew we'd probably bring him down to 120. I heard Dr. Kelly's whine (why did I always hear him as a whine?), "He doesn't need all that weight for a wheelchair existence."

David's attitude seemed pretty good, but I was worried about him. He was asking more and more questions about why we were standing him in the parallel bars. I thought he should be told that he wasn't going to walk again. I thought it was time.

When I arrived I headed straight for Dr. Kelly's office. He put his pipe down and looked up at me above his half-glasses. I always felt like I was bothering him. I told him I thought we had made the wrong decision at the rehab conference about not telling David yet. He stood up, and although I was still standing, I remember feeling as if I'd just sat down.

"Leave that to me, Ruth. He needs the hope at this point. You're doing an excellent job with him. He adores you. Don't take away the hope. He'll adjust."

I dragged myself to the clinic. David was waiting, and I pushed him to the parallel bars. I could spit nails today, as my dad used to say. David was surly, too. I proceeded, ignoring his rudeness but nurturing the festering in my own spirit. Once we were up, he hissed, "Are you ever going to stop making me do this nonsense? I feel like a dancing bear on my hind legs. Of course, one difference. They can stand up. (Pause) Damn it! How much time do we have left? (I don't answer. Another pause. I can tell he is going to attack from another angle.) The only good part is that you hold me so tight. Mm Baby. Baby. Baby. Too bad I can't feel anything. How does it feel hugging a circus animal for an hour a day?"

I smiled, but my heart iced over like the thick frost clinging to the edges of the clinic window. I was trying to *help* him. Did he really think I enjoyed hugging his ugly body? I *despised* him. I wanted to drop him on the floor right then and there, and he wouldn't be able to get up by himself. Or maybe I'd take him into Dr. Kelly's office and drop him on the floor in front of Dr. Kelly and walk out.

DECEMBER 22

Things sometimes get really hard. I dreaded treating David because . . . well, because the anger had dissipated into something that hurt so much and seemed so useless, and at the same time I really did believe that David had placed a heavy rock of hope around my neck. Or was it that I had pinned hope to his sticky shirt that always smelled of body oil and sweat?

We were locked in an embrace on a tightrope.

Sometimes these days we went through the parallel bars part of the treatment day with very little conversation, or only strained conversation. Finally today he asked, in an unusually loud voice, "How much do I weigh anyway?"

"The nurses say you're down to 160."

"160 pounds. I guess they're trying to starve me so I can roll around in the wheelchair better."

I paused, trying to choose my next words carefully. "Has Dr. Kelly been talking to you about that?"

"About what?"

"About the wheelchair?"

"No. But who's kidding who? I ain't walking again, Ruth."

"Well, as you know, we've been working to see if there is any chance of your being able to walk at all."

In a much smaller voice he replied, "You can save your time, Ruth. I ain't walking again and we both know it."

I felt tears welling up in my eyes. David noticed before I could turn my head away. The orderlies noticed. One looked at me sympathetically, the other averted his eyes.

"It's OK," David said. "We tried."

He cocked his head toward the Kleenex box on the table. "I'd get you one myself," he said with a half smile, "if I could."

Without my command the three of us lowered David back into the wheelchair. The orderlies disappeared. He and I sat, in a long silence.

I used the same Kleenex to wipe his eyes.

JANUARY 10

I welcomed the week of vacation. Even with a howling wind chill, the lake is a mother that restores. Somehow the knowledge that David and I shared was freeing, and when I returned it was with renewed vigor for my work.

Ken said that Dr. Kelly wanted to see me right away. I was

still too relaxed from the holidays to experience the feeling of dread that a visit to his office usually evoked.

I stood. He never asked anyone to sit.

"Thanks for coming. I know you are busy. Did you enjoy your holiday? Good." He hesitated, a well-placed pause for effect. Then, in his physician's voice, "Was there a reason you chose to tell David he would not walk again, just before you left for Christmas?"

I stammered, feeling guilty, "Actually, he told me, Dr. Kelly."

"*He* told *you*, Ruth? I think that you and David are getting too attached. It does happen with young therapists. I'm thinking that maybe I should transfer him to someone else. What do you think?"

For the first time ever, my fear of Dr. Kelly was totally displaced by seething. I tried to keep an even voice. "I think we're doing fine. And I think it would be hard on him at this point to be transferred to someone else."

"He was depressed when you were gone last week on vacation."

"Is that so unusual? Besides, he was left here at Christmas. I'd be depressed too. I thought about him, and Mr. Kavanaugh, and Joyce and *all* the . . ."

"Well. It's not good for patients here to get so attached. It does them a real disservice."

"You know, I really would like to continue to work with David. I feel like we're just starting to make some progress."

Dr. Kelly was mulling it over, or pretending to. After an interminable period of time he said, looking past me out the window, "Well, do remember our conversation, then."

JANUARY 15

The January-to-springtime period was going to be hard on David. We discussed it in our staff rehabilitation conference. The psychologist said he would step up his efforts to get David to talk about his diving experience, a move David had not made to any of us. His girlfriend, Jane, a cheerleader, would be coming less often during the winter months because of icy roads and the hockey season. This beautiful, green-eyed, black-haired teenager seemed devoted, but I sensed she was growing weary. The able-bodied grow weary. His buddies had grown weary.

David was resting between the strengthening exercises we were attempting for the small return he was getting in his shoulders. Without warning the drumbeats rolled and the parade began to march out of David's soul.

"I like ran the winning touchdown. Jim my brother—"

"Of course. I know your brother. He came to the clinic last week when you were having your treatment. The big guy in the cutoff teeshirt."

"That's right. That's him. Yeah. Jim. God I love Jim. He's a beast."

"A beast?"

"Well, I call him a beast because he's the only one around bigger than me." (David laughed. Silence. His eyes went blank, then watery.) "That is, before . . . (his voice trailed off and he didn't finish the sentence).

"Anyway. Jim is hollering loud. Above all the other guys. I can hear his voice and I'm running like hell . . . So. Afterwards Jim and Jane and I . . . Jane . . . (he goes silent again). Jane. Did you know Jane brought me that goddamn football for Christmas? All the team sent messages on the football . . . So. Where was I? After the game the three of us we went out to a friend's place on the outskirts of town. I had a few beers you know. I felt like a million bucks . . . I dived. I dived into three goddamn feet of water. When I hit I knew. I just knew. I thought, 'I'm dead. An animal stuck in the muck. I'm already dead.'"

"Did you really think, 'An animal stuck in the muck'"?

"I think so. I had an idea of something like that. The next thing I can remember I was staring at the ceiling. I was a head. Just a head. Only a head. The rest of my body was still back there in the muck at the bottom of Mouse River."

"Do you feel like your body has come back to be with your head?"

He had been looking off into space during the last few sentences. With my question his eyes swung back to mine with such force that it appeared his whole paralyzed body had moved toward me. "Would you?"

My gaze hit the floor and I was silent for a long time.

"I don't know, David."

JANUARY 30

My post-Christmas energy continued through the bleak January days. David was adjusting to the wheelchair. He was making good progress in his shoulder exercises and a nagging kidney infection had cleared up. He was talking to the psychologist on a regular basis.

"Raise your head, kid. It's Monday!" I chided. "You been on a weekend binge or something?"

He continued to sit, slumped over, scowling. I noticed how diminutive his figure now seemed, but when he spoke his voice still roared. "No. But I need a drink."

"What do you mean, you need a drink?"

"It doesn't matter anymore. All those weights. The pulleys. Just get me outta here."

He couldn't move any part of his body, but I felt as if he had physically thrown something at the wall, or at me. The alarms went off in my spirit.

"David! *What's the matter?*"

His shoulders sagged lower and I saw the flaps of skin on his chin and belly . . . Eighty pounds lighter too quickly for his young skin to keep up with his diminishing bulk. He raised his head, barely, and whispered hoarsely from somewhere way back in his throat, or life, "Jane is going to marry Jim."

For the first time ever, I was without words with David. He looked straight into my eyes, locked in that moment of recognition that we had both lost our footing and were falling.

There is a lion in the Las Vegas MGM Hotel lobby. He is not chained or caged. They put that look in his eyes, too. He knew

that whatever anyone did to him, he would never move from
that spot on his own power.

FEBRUARY 25

I visited him daily at his bedside to do passive range of motion exercises. Some of the nurses and one occupational therapist were as "attached" as I. We agreed to keep a kind of vigil. Three, almost four weeks had passed with him looking blankly at everyone. Some days I wanted to stop. I was scared.

MARCH 10

It was Monday morning. (It was always Monday morning.) When I went to his room at mid-morning, he had his face to the wall. I wondered with some irritation who turned him in that position. I said his name gently.

"I'm on strike today. Go away!"

I jumped back, shocked at the energy in his voice after so many almost lifeless days. My irritation shifted from the staff to David.

"What do you *mean*, you're on strike?" I said, struggling to regain a stance that paralleled his sudden revival. "You've been on strike for weeks. David, if you don't start doing something, they are going to send you home. I don't want that to happen. You'll be lonely." (Silence.)

"What's up, David?" I asked, feeling more tentative again.

"I don't want to be lonely! I just want to be alone!"

APRIL 13

For over a month David did his work of solitude. He agreed to go to occupational therapy, but that was the only "real" rehabilitation he had been doing since his bad news about Jim and Jane. Even so, the rest of us were more hopeful. We imagined that *he* was beginning to re-emerge, or emerge.

His parents came more often. Not Jim. Not Jane. He was starting to talk about going home. The vocational rehabilitation counselors explored the possibility of adapting a tractor that he might be able to operate, to help his dad on the farm. Most of us dismissed that idea as impossible. Most of us predicted that he would be in a nursing home, or dead, within a year after his discharge.

MAY 18 (note from my journal)
Next week several of the therapists, including myself, will take some of the young people at the center to a traveling circus that is coming to town. That should be some undertaking, but we will try to do it.

MAY 20
David, in an offhanded, embarrassed gesture, came into the clinic with a bread board balanced on his knees. A product of his work in occupational therapy.

"Something to remember me by," he said.

I saw Kathleen, an occupational therapist, framed in the distant doorway behind him, a smile on her face.

MAY 24 (note from my journal)
It is one of the first real summer nights of the year. Sultry, the heavy air of August, but it's only May. I can't sleep. Is it the heat?

There were eight of them and ten of us. When we arrived at the circus grounds, we realized we would have to navigate a large plowed field to get to the circus tent.

With the help of an orderly I pushed David's wheelchair across the field, laughing and sweating all the way.

As our entourage made their way across the field, a crowd of people who had been watching the clowns and buying balloons and touching the elephants began to watch us. They lined up in silent awe as we continued our journey.

Just as I was pushing David's chair through the door of the circus tent a small, loose-jawed, redheaded boy not more than seven, his eyes as round as doorknobs, took a step forward and placed his hand on David's shoulder.

"You guys been in a *wreck* or something?" he said.

David tried, unsuccessfully to turn his head toward the small boy.

"Geez! He's alive!" The boy bolted back.

I heard David say, ever so softly, as the parade of wheelchairs and walkers continued toward their special place in front of the first row of bleachers, "Yeah. A wreck. Or something."

POSTLUDE

Sometimes, when I remember David being hoisted into the transport van for his ride home, the electric wheelchair is a cage holding a once-wild beast captive in a ridiculously bolt-upright position. At other times his figure simply rises, being lighter than air itself. At those times, he soars out of sight to heights or depths known only to other mythical beings of college textbooks and, now, dreams.

If you ask the people at the rehabilitation center, they will say David died, in a nursing home, not one but two years later. Kidney failure.

I still use the bread board.

WITNESS

Veneta Masson

Sunday
after church
under a sleeve of summer sky
we walk up the alley
called Wiltberger Street,
look down
at the bloodstained cement.

He was fourteen
on just another
hip hop high top
Saturday
in the hood when
somebody put his lights out—
semiautomatic.

The people who live
on the alley
behind brick facades
won't talk
but lock up their kids
for the weekend.
They could be next.

I want to kneel
in this stagnant pool
of spent rage,
smear the blood all over
my face, my clothes
and wander like Cain
through the city and say

Look at me and see
what I have seen.

But I don't.
I stay where I am,
nursing the wounds
that never heal for want
of the capacity to feel—
like ulcers on a sole
bereft of sensation.

What balm is there
in this violent Gilead
to make the wounded whole?
I know no cure
and all I have is breath
a voice
and memory—

    a memory
    a voice.

Connection
and
Disconnection

MAGGIE JONES
Veneta Masson

Just
who do you think you are, Maggie Jones,
following me home from work
insinuating yourself into my evening
shading my thoughts?

Just
who do you think you are
lying flat as a pancake in the middle of your bed
your world ranged around you in brown paper bags?

(Rather like a dead pharaoh in his tomb, I'd say,
buried with all his treasure.)

So you fell one day and had to be taken
    to the hospital.
You didn't break any bones, after all,
You came home in a taxi
climbed the steep flight of stairs to your room
took to your bed and stayed there.
That was three years ago, Maggie,
Three years with only one thing to look forward to—
    livin'.

I'm here by the hand of the Lord, you always say
    when I come
though the hand of the Lord didn't smite the rat
    that bit your foot
    that cold winter day last year
    as it foraged in your sheets for bread and jelly.
I guess it'll be all right,
    you said in your genteel way
    looking up at me with soft doe eyes as I dressed
    the wound that brought us together.

Why don't you go to a home? we ask, shocked
    to see the condition you're in
    (the church ladies, the social worker,
    your niece, your nephew, and I).
Because I still have my right mind,
    you say simply.
    A nursing home is no place
    for someone who still has their mind.

But it's not safe here, we say
    (the church ladies, the social worker,
    your niece, your nephew, and I).
Don't you know they shoot drugs
    and people in this neighborhood?
I've never been bothered,
    you say, matter-of-factly.

What about fire? we say
    (the church ladies, the social worker,
    your niece, your nephew, and I).
You'd be burned alive in your bed.
There was a fire once, and the fireman carried me out.
I own my home and I own my grave plot
    and I plan to go from one to the other
    when the Lord calls me,
    you say quietly, clutching a packet
    of long white envelopes.

But now your gas is cut off
    until you come up with $700.
You're lucky it's not freezing and there's an electric
    coffeemaker we can use
    to heat water to wash you.
I guess the money will come from somewhere,
    you say, looking at me steadily.

And Meals on Wheels has cut you off because it's a bad
    neighborhood to begin with and then

the front door fell off its hinges
onto the Meals on Wheels delivery lady.
I guess there's enough food in the United States
    to feed me,
    you say, looking at me knowingly.

And they've taken away your homemaker because they say
    you need more care
    than the agency can give.
I guess things will work out,
    you say, looking at me trustingly.

How can you lie there and say serenely you guess
    things will work out?
    Your room is cold
    your sheets are soaked with urine
    your skin is bleeding from bedsores
    you don't know where your next meal is coming from
    you're a poor old lady
        hidden away
        in a falling-down house
        in a no-good neighborhood.
    And you have expectations?

You told your niece not to worry about you
    the nurse was coming.
Hey, Maggie Jones, don't wait for me, don't count on me.
    I'll bathe you
    dress your wounds
    treat your minor ailments
    even do your laundry and bring you food
    once in a while.

But save you?
God alone—the hand of the Lord—can save you.

I see you now in my mind's eye and wonder
    as I sit

after dinner
in my warm house
on a safe street
in a good neighborhood
Just
who do you think you are, Maggie Jones?

(originally published in *Just Who* [Washington, D.C.: Crossroad Health Ministry, 1993])

DEHISCENCE

Amy Haddad

You have come unstitched.

Holes appear on your threadbare abdomen.
Tunnels develop and connect bowel, liver, pancreas.
Enzymes ooze out and digest your skin,
no matter how hard we try to stem the flow.
Mounds of dressings,
miles of tape—a jerry-rigged system to
hold together our mistakes.
The stench is overwhelming, ever present
reminding everyone, but especially you,
that you have come undone.

Since I cannot bear your suffering,
since the truth is too horrible to grasp,
since I can offer you nothing else,
I clean you up.
I wash your face,
brush your teeth,
comb your hair,
turn you gently on your side,
push soiled linens away,
roll clean sheets under you,
remove layers and layers of damp, disgusting dressings,
and replace them with new dressings and tape.

Since I am helpless in the face of your tragedy,
I give you the certainty and calmness of my motions,
the competence and comfort of my touch
as I smooth the top sheet over my work.
Done.

For a few pristine moments, we allow ourselves
to be caught in the illusion of your wholeness.

(originally published in *Between the Heartbeats: Poetry and Prose by Nurses*,
edited by C. Davis and J. Schaefer [Iowa City: University of Iowa Press,
1995], p. 86)

TICKET TO CHRISTMAS

Veneta Masson

That day, that Christmas Eve last year,
I went to work as usual, but full of expectation.
I went to the clinic expecting Christmas
to happen to me. I thought I knew what it would be—
most probably a patient and a poignant interruption
in the flow of everyday. There might be merriment
or tears. There would be touch. I'd touch
and let myself be touched by Christmas.

All morning patients came and went.
Some laughed. One wept.
I touched them and was touched in turn.
But none of them was Christmas.
By afternoon, I knew there was something more
I needed to do. I'd go to the market
across the street, buy cookies and punch
and set them out in the waiting room
like a child making ready for Santa.

There wasn't much time, patients were waiting.
I threw on my coat and ran out the door
just in time to catch a green light.
But a voice called out from the P Street side
of the liquor store. Christmas had been there
waiting for me. Startled, I stopped,
missed the light, stepped backwards
up, onto the curb. There wasn't much time.
Patients were waiting. I deeply resented
the interruption even though I knew who it was.

Christmas was black, fifty or so, wearing
an Orioles' baseball cap. He swayed a little
but didn't reek and started to speak as if

he had something to say I needed to hear.
I'm homeless, he said, and then he told
how long ago he'd prayed to God to show him
how it was to live on the streets, but just today
he'd been telling God he'd had enough.
Where will you spend the night? I asked.
In the shelter at Second and D, he said.

He wanted to give me a present. I wanted
to make the light. I knew he was Christmas
but I was uneasy and wanted to be on my way.
Wait, he said and started to empty his
pockets into my hands: a red and green bag
with a pair of white socks, a lottery ticket
he made me scratch while he halted the search
(we didn't win), folded papers, a tattered
social security card, and so on down to the lint
in the seams until at last he found it.

"Admit One" is what it said. A ticket to
the Christmas gala the city puts on for
down and outs. Take it, he said. I've seen
it all—the stars, the food, the fancy decorations.
But don't go dressed like you are right now.
Go home and change into something a homeless
person might wear so you can feel just what
it's like. You get my meaning, don't you, Miss?

I waited for the hustle. It never came.
He never asked for money or a date.
I put the ticket into my pocket and left him
when the light turned green. As I made my way
to the grocery store I heard his voice
behind me once more. Miss! he called.
Remember that's my ticket. Remember
that ticket's my Christmas gift to you.

EVALUATIONS

Lynne Willett

Christmas is a special time in the Neonatal Intensive Care Unit. Sure we put up all the requisite decor, the trappings of a celebration none of the families can feel. We all pretend a cheeriness in the hopes of raising spirits—theirs and ours. But the real meaning of this time of year lies in the Christmas cards and pictures we receive. This is the reckoning, our end-of-the-year evaluation, our bonus or our comeuppance.

Each year we anxiously await those cards and pore through them, reading between the lines, trying to find the truth—did the marriage survive? Is the mother coping OK? Is Grandma raising the teenager's baby? More important still, how is the child *really?* We scrutinize those two-dimensional pictures to try and make a 3-D image. How much does that child see? Is he making his milestones? Does she look all right?

We have learned all too painfully over the years that babies who look normal when they go home from the hospital are not measure of success. It is through these cards and pictures that we glimpse the true fruits of our labor, the good and the bad. This is where we receive the final thanks and gratification, making our work worthwhile. It is also where we see our bitterest shortcomings. Reviewing these cards and letters is an unspoken ritual here. They are placed on a bulletin board for all to see and to educate the families now here about what is expected of them. They can see what it means to all of us.

Thinking about these Christmas scenes reminds me of the only time my grandmother came to visit me at work. She was in her seventies and had heard often of the NICU. Grandma had grown up in rural Nebraska and had premature twins of her own during the Depression on Valentine's Day. I had loved hearing the story of how she delivered them at home, with the family doctor coming to help. She had no idea there were two babies. She delivered the boy first and cried when the doctor told her there was another baby still to come. They were both puny little things that the doctor guessed weighed about three pounds each, as he held them up in his hands. He didn't think they would survive and left them in the care of my great grandmother, who placed them in boxes by the fire with a hot water bottle and heated bricks to keep them warm. The smaller, second twin kept turning blue, so my grandmother and great grandmother took turns watching over them. Each time the babies would stop breathing, Grandma would clear their throats and bend them up and down like an accordion to make them gasp. For days they were fed with eyedroppers until they were strong enough to nipple alone. Many years later the second twin became my mother.

So I was bursting with pride when I toured the NICU with Grandmother, knowing how impressed she would be by all the equipment and the tiny occupants of the isolettes. I showed how much everything had changed since her babies were born and what we could do for them now. She didn't say much as I bubbled on in my excitement to have her at last understand what I did for a living. As the final coup de grâce, I showed her the bulletin board with the pictures of the NICU "graduates." My grandmother sniffed and turned to me saying, "They all look retarded to me."

THE THINGS YOU DO
Kelly Jennings Olson

Abe walks by the girl's head, leading. He cradles her jaw, thrusting it forward, to keep her airway open. Even as near as we are to the emergency room, we stop whenever Abe hears a gurgle in her throat. When he says "now," Marilyn pulls back the oxygen mask and I suction the blood and fluid. Holding her head still, opening her mouth, and keeping her airway clear; these are awkward things to do, rolling down a hospital corridor.

Right now, they are the most important things.

Her name is Mamie. She is five years old, her father told us, while crouching beside us in the furrow.

One of the ER nurses, Evelyn, touches my shoulder. I smell the soap she just used, and rubbing alcohol. "Mamie Owens," I explain. "Age five. Tractor accident. Head and abdominal injuries. BP is 90 over 60. Pulse weak and 140 beats per minute."

"Mamie is my cousin's child," she breathes, and then I remember. This is a small town I have come to live in.

Abe tells her about the IV he started, the solution, and the drip rate. Evelyn nods without looking away from Mamie. She steps into the procession, takes over my task, and hurries everyone toward the sterile room where she will unwrap and survey the person we've found and carried.

"She slipped off the tractor seat beside me," he said, "and she went under the tire." He paced back and forth, twisting his cap in his hands. While I wrapped the blood pressure cuff snug, he knelt beside me, squeezing my arm. I patted his hand, looked into his eyes, and said, "I'm doing what I can, but you need to step back so I can work, okay?" He nodded, but he didn't move, and his eyes never left his daughter. I put the stethoscope in my ears and tried to hear her swooshing blood pressure beats over the din of his anguish.

I lean against the painted cinder block wall, next to a local artist's cartoony painting of a barn, two grazing horses, and a hay rake. I look down at my hands. They're trembling.

I remember a story Abe told us once at an ambulance meeting. A child fell off a tractor while his father was plowing. The back tire rolled over his head, but the ground was soft and the child was only bruised.

The fluorescent lights hum to me that this is an often-told story.

I shove my hands into my jacket pockets and walk to the emergency room, in case I am needed. But the other crew members, all volunteers like me, one by one step back. We don't know what to do in such a large space. A whole room. Enamel cupboards, freestanding gooseneck lamps, and chairs. Mirrored halogen lights overhead. Nothing's rocking side to side, either. No siren. Our compact, abbreviated motions are designed, scaled, and practiced to fit in the back of an ambulance, or the spaces between beds and nightstands, or in stairwells where someone has fallen. In here we're like unswaddled babies, startled by the range of our motion.

I hear Dr. Blau say he's calling a Carelift helicopter for Mamie. "Beyond me," he mutters. "Internal injuries, and head trauma, too. She needs a pediatric trauma specialist, and we're losing our 'golden hour.' Watch for her father. A tall guy, red hair." He's coaching me, since I just moved to town two years ago and don't know everybody. But we work at accident scenes with parents sitting on our backs, demanding, grieving. I never forget the parents.

When I see Mamie's father burst in, almost not waiting for the doors to part like Red Sea water, when I see him almost swoop into the glass like a mesmerized starling into a picture window, I take him by the arm and sit with him.

He stares at my shirt. I look down and see it's smeared with Mamie's blood. "It looks like more than it is," I say, then change the subject. "Dr. Blau's calling for a helicopter to take her to Sioux Falls." He nods, but he's still staring at my shirt and starts to cry. I try to zip my jacket over the red blotch, but he puts out a hand to stop me. He wants to see.

The ground was soft, freshly plowed for planting where I knelt beside Mamie. I hope.

Abe walks up to us. He holds out a cup of coffee, steaming. "Gary," he says.

The father looks up and takes the cup. "My God, Abe, what have I done?"

Abe shakes his head and squats down in front of Gary. "Not you. It was an accident."

"It was my fault. And she wants to be a farmer," Gary mumbles. "She wants to be like me."

Abe notices my shirt and says, "It's okay, I'll stay with him."

As I walk by, Dr. Blau looks up at me over his clipboard and swallows like something's stuck in his throat, but his voice is flat, professional. "We need a landing area for the helicopter." Although the hospital administrator doesn't approve, we have to use the parking lot for a pad. There's a field nearby that we're supposed to use. But it's not quite level, and the dust and chaff blow so high that you hate to land a helicopter in that garbage if you don't have to. Why risk that?

I stop by the ER door and ask Marilyn if she'll go out with me to clear the parking lot and wave in the helicopter. She hesitates. "I feel like if I stand here, maybe it'll help," she says. "You know, I had her in Sunday school last year. She used more red glitter and glue than any child I've ever seen. Always red on red on red."

I lean around Marilyn to look in. Between two nurses I see a small hand with an IV stuck into it, taped to a board. That and a tangle of brown hair at the head of the examining table. Mamie Owens. Is she in my daughter Justine's kindergarten class? Is it her mother who works at SuperMart? Blonde?

Marilyn and I walk down the hall, reviewing. "It's getting dark, so we'll need to make sure the area's well-lit, free of sticks and trash" and "the lights can't blind the pilot as he tries to land" and "we have to note the wind, and spot any wires, or poles." We say it for each other, like a litany, as we pass between the automatic doors.

The dusk outside reminds me of the new Lenten banner at Willow Bend Church—thick, like wool or felt, and purple, like Mamie's lips when I knelt down beside her behind the tractor tire.

Marilyn clears the asphalt of a few cottonwood branches that came down in last night's early-spring hailstorm. I pitch loose stones into the field nearby and wonder, how did I get into this? Abe's wife, Marilyn, is the person who talked me into emergency medical technician training, then into volunteering, when I came to town because of my husband's job. She's volunteered for fifteen years. She's seen a lot, so I ask her, "What do you think?"

Marilyn shakes her head, muttering, "I hope . . ."

I understand. "I hope" is what we say when it's bad, and all we can do is pray someone will make it. There's no way of telling when they won't, but you just get this feeling. Even when you feel it, you never say it. Not even if you're having to do all the heartbeats and breaths for them.

Maybe it's because they might hear you. Unconscious people, dying people, hear everything. And people often know when they're going to die. Sometimes they say, "I'm not gonna make it." Sometimes they ask, just to be sure, "I'm gonna die, aren't I?"

In training I learned to answer, "We're doing what we can to help you."

Maybe it's stubbornness, or an act of faith, but you never admit it until the person's dead, silent, flat-line on the monitor and the doctor pronounces it final.

Ask anybody.

"I'll try the parking lot lights." Marilyn goes inside the hospital door and flips a switch. Yellow cones shine down around the lampposts, but don't do much to illuminate the center of the square.

Marilyn's looking, thinking, and I call out, "They're coming from the south, heading north. I'll move the ambulance outside the lot and shine the headlights across the pavement, east to west." Marilyn waves, okay. After taking the garden hose and wetting down the dusty asphalt, she unclips the portable radio from her belt and talks to the helicopter pilot, who's already within radio range. She warns him about the telephone wires on the west side and the gusts of wind from the north. As I walk to the ambulance, I hear the pilot's voice crackling static.

Mamie was wearing a Bart Simpson T-shirt. I had to cut it with my crash scissors so I could palpate her ribs. But I cut along the seams, so it could be repaired. I hope.

Switching on the ambulance radio, I can understand the pilot now. Through the windshield I see the doctor and nurses and Mamie's father huddled around the ambulance cot in the glassed-in hospital entry, standing back so they don't set off the door sensor. They won't come out until the helicopter's landed. Marilyn's voice, louder than the pilot's, comes over the radio, "Can we load her rotors hot? The patient's critical."

"Ten-four."

I shut off the radio and walk around to the side, looking south. Then I see it. A white dragonfly with blinking red eyes darts over the town toward us. By the time I can hear it, I'm afraid that it's not going to see us, that the pilot will pass over and end up in Brookings. It's going that fast. Has this pilot been here before? We've only called the helicopter once. It's a new thing for us.

I hurry to the hospital door and wait, peering around my jacket sleeve. I hear flying gravel ka-tinking against the glass doors. The helicopter floats down, down, and settles like an old aunt onto a couch. Easy.

Oh, he's good at that. He lands that thing like he grew up down the street and is just back for a visit. Maybe he did, and is. Dr. Blau flips a corner of the blanket over Mamie's face. Once the helicopter's firm on the ground, the hospital doors open. They all hurry out, shielding Mamie with their bodies and making the cot look like a centipede. Nurses hold IV bags up in the air and everyone cringes, knees bent to avoid the rapid, invisible rotors. The pilot barely slows the engine to save time for Mamie. Rotors hot. The noise is like wind and thunder and hail on a roof, all at once.

The pavement's rough and the cot's aluminum tubing vibrates under my hands. Beside the helicopter, we unbuckle the straps that hold Mamie. On the count of three, all our hands, one by another, by another, lift up the long backboard. As it passes out of our reach, we touch the wood like a benediction, and I hear Marilyn yell, "Go on, Mamie." Someone, I don't know who, reaches over and ruffles Mamie's hair. It could have been any of us, or all.

I realize what I couldn't admit before, that Mamie's hair blows in that rotor wind the same golden brown as Justine's. Yes, but for some grace or random honor it could be my child lying there. But there is a greater thing, more fearsome . . . by some sticky web, some tangling of community, I've stumbled here into Hayden Corners, Mamie not only could be, but is, mine. And Abe's and Marilyn's and Evelyn's. And the drawstring-cinching of that owning and risk makes my legs feel like water, until I reach over for Marilyn's arm, grabbing the slick red poly-ester of her ambulance jacket, and she grasps my hand. She must know, surely she does, because she looks at me and her eyes say, "welcome."

Straining to make out that pale face through the curved glass, we pull the light, bounding cot over the blacktop, away from the helicopter. Our eyes don't want to let her go. A nurse is bending over Mamie, like inside a fishbowl. The pilot and one Carelift nurse secure the side door, then get in the front.

The engine and rotors pick up their pitch one octave and we have to look away, now that we're back out where the wind snatches our breath and throws dirt in our eyes. We peer through slits between our fingers, though.

The copter rises, bobs, then levitates, and I think how Mamie would be glad, how any five-year-old girl would love to be part of such a trick, hovering so high a magician could pass a hoop around her, end to end. No wires. I hope someone gets a chance to tell her how she looks, hang-ing between the earth and clouds, and what a wonder she is to all of us. I hope I get to tell her. Then she's gone.

We all stand there, straining our eyes into the sky, which has hardened from purple to charcoal gray. Then we look down at the pavement, air-swept clean. A nurse's aide marches up to Gary, says she's done on her shift, and she'll drive him to Sioux Falls. She's jingling her keys and guiding Gary like a blind man to her car.

Marilyn and I walk over to the ambulance, squinting against the headlights. We climb in to get things organized. I list the equipment we need to get back from inside the hospital: the cardiac monitor, blood pressure cuff, O2 bottle, and portable suction kit. I guess I lost my penlight out in the field. Marilyn sighs and snaps a clean sheet in the air over the cot, then tucks the edges underneath.

Back inside the hospital, after we've restocked and parked the ambulance, Marilyn says she'll fill out the trip report with Abe.

"Just sign here, and go home to your kids," she tells me. "It's getting late. We'll finish."

Just inside the emergency room door, I see that shirt crumpled on the floor. Bart Simpson pop-eyed smiling at me. Reckless, plucky rascal. Blood on his caption balloon. I fold it, blood side in, and stuff it in my jacket pocket. Marilyn's watching me from the nurses' station, so I explain, "I have something that might take the stain out. I'll stitch up the sides."

Marilyn nods at me, because these are the things you do.

Just ask anybody.

SECRETS

Kate Brown

Secrets. There's no such thing as secrets in this town. Everybody knows everything, or so they think. That's the way I figure it at least and then just carry on with life like it was an open book. Might as well, anyway. It's strange though, because most people are like me—we just keep to ourselves. So how is it that anybody knows anything at all, since nobody seems to be doing the telling? Or so we say.

Could be it's the woodwork and the church pews that tell. Maybe the coffee mugs in the cafe—that's a sure bet for spreading gossip if anything was doing it. Really though, I think it's just that we've lived so long with each other here that we see things, feel things, we know things, without talking about it—like how you can notice the itch on the inside of your own arm. Without paying any attention to it with your mind, you scratch just where the itch is. You may not even notice you're scratching, but you are.

One time when my cousin's wife had "female" cancer she didn't tell a soul, except her husband. Cancer's one thing nobody wants to talk about, like if you did it would take off, building like a dark cloud on a summer day when a storm grows up from nowhere. You know that old saying, don't you: "Don't trouble trouble"? That means pretty plainly don't bring it up. Just let it lie quiet. That's what we were taught.

And her, she's got it double with the female thing because that's every woman's privacy. That's what we learned to call it even, "private parts," you know? She didn't tell anyone except Stan; I know that for a fact. So how did the preacher know to ask us to pray for her cancer surgery a week later?

Whispers, that's how. Whispers through the fields, up the aisles in the grocery store, in and out of the mailboxes at the post office. Whispers, and nobody talking. No, nobody said a word, but word spread, just like how you know about the itch down along the inside of your arm. It's like we're connected, like we're some kind of living thing, like that coral reef I saw on TV out by Australia.

Impossible, you say? Maybe, maybe not. There was that other time too. The time we all knew we needed to get down to Merlie's place after the tornado. And sure enough, the whole side of their house was nowhere to be seen and we all just stood there looking, kind of embarrassed and surprised to be there. How'd we get there? I ask you.

THE NURSE'S TASK

Cortney Davis

When I pluck the suture
or pack the ulcer with gauze,
it becomes my task
to introduce rage to this body

that calls me, *nurse, nurse,*
as if my hands were gold.
First I cradle the body
like a mother rocks.

I lean close
and let it memorize my face.
Then I begin.
First, something subtle.

A hasty scrape.
An accidental pinch
as if I might thrust needle
down to bone. The body

raises its hands in disbelief.
This is nothing. I thread veins
with catheters of fire,
I change morphine to milk.

When the body asks *why?*
I am silent. When the body
whines, I act bored
and turn away. If sleep comes

I sneak in and shake the body

until, angry and squinty-eyed,
it rises on its elbow
and stares at me,

at last understanding
that the flesh is everything—
we live only
in its narrow bed.

This then is the body
I love—the one
that laughs down death's trumpet.
The one that escapes.

(first appeared in an earlier version in the *International Journal of Arts-Medicine* [Fall 1991])

NURSE AS ANGEL OF MERCY

Cortney Davis

She has seen the artificial eye
afloat in a glass and the wig
in the bald lady's room. Undisturbed,
she directs her flashlight beam
onto each languid face.
Patients twitch or feel a breeze.
If they wake they find
an empty room, nurses' voices

distant as a mother's song.
The Angel, full-breasted and fat,
is busy checking, tucking.
She wipes her hands on her skirts,
enters the room of her favorite—
the boy spun like a chrysalis
in cocoons of tubes and stainless wires,
drifting to the *blink-tap* of pumps,

the syncope of bellows.
He dreams he is face up in a rowboat,
her light a single red sun
wormed through his lids. She bends
to kiss his lips, she
plucks him from his tethers,
hoists him like a sack.
He dreams his boat is rocked by waves.

Tubes snap. The red-eyed pump goes blind.
Doctors hurry into the room,
flail the boy until he is blue

and they are spent.
They cover the shell of his face.
Down the hall, limping, out of breath,
the Angel runs, her favorite
dancing on her back like awkward wings.

(first appeared in *Literature and Medicine* [Spring 1992])

BELLE

Claudia Peyton

No one will ever know just how long she wandered the streets in that timeless existence of having no place to go and no one to meet her there. In that emotional vacuum of confusion that allows a person to wander for days, weeks, and years without direction.

To have no distinctions between the night and the day or between purpose and none, to have no sense of self, no roles to fill.

What must time become in this space of skid row existence?

Is there any way to know the inner dimensions of a meaningless, fearful existence with no comfort but the withdrawal from others, or structure, or maybe society, to a space of wandering aimlessly, confused, taken advantage of, through a threatening maze of city streets?

If psychosis isn't a part of beginning this wandering journey, it must certainly be the outcome.

She slept by the back door of the Women's Center for many nights, in the alley near the dumpster. She wandered during the day and would return to sleep. She would not come in for meals or a shower; the alley was her only port in this storm.

We waited, watching patiently as she fought against trusting us.

I remember allowing myself to see her for the first time— really looking at her, even though months had passed since her arrival at the back door step. Now I believe that it was my own pain of knowing that she was there and not open to help that prevented my attending to her. There had been a distance that I wasn't able to acknowledge.

She wore thick dark eye shadow and covered her nearly shaved head with a turban made of old scarves. She wore layers of skirts and blouse upon blouse, summer and winter. She was not a young woman, yet not frail. Her teeth were black with decay and she moved very slowly and gazed as if looking toward a faraway place.

Once inside, she wandered through the center, never sitting, always moving or standing very still, listening to herself, motionless, staring sometimes for a very long time.

She often went to the desk drawer and took scissors. She would then disappear into the corner, reach under her turban of scarves and cut her hair and then eat it.

I wondered what this ritual meant to her.

Even with this madness, she had a certain style, a uniqueness all her own. Though her language could not be understood, as it was garbled and fragmented, she had a look, a constant sense of gypsy-like style and color.

I remember our first face-to-face encounter: the trash can was very heavy and I needed to move it through the back door and empty it into the dumpster. She was there in the kitchen, where she had been sweeping in one place for a very long time, wanting to help, yet immobile. I couldn't lift the can up the steps, and everyone was busy except Belle. I motioned to her for help, as I knew she was watching me carefully out of the corner of her eye. She stopped sweeping. She stared and spoke in words that were familiar yet had no order or meaning I could understand. She let the broom fall as she moved toward me, she took the other side of the trash can and lifted it. I knew in my heart that this was a beginning.

The two of us moved slowly, the garbage almost too heavy to carry. We spoke of our frustration through brief glances. Breathing heavily, we lifted the can, struggling, depending on each other not to let go. We did it. After we eased the can to the ground, we smiled at our accomplishment and went inside. She returned to her sweeping, the first meaningful activity since her long journey to this place of safety.

Belle spent many days sweeping in one place while the rest of us cleaned the center. It was important to her to be a part of what others were doing, and eventually she added a new activity. She washed cups from lunchtime until dinner. Washing one, drying it, then walking the length of the center to place the cup next to the coffee pots, which were on the table near the front door. She didn't seem to notice the time, or maybe she wanted to savor the moments of doing something to show her gratitude for having found this safe place. She was coming back from a long journey and each week seemed better than the one before, a little closer.

For many months she continued to keep a distance from the other ladies, who were gathered in small groups playing cards or Scrabble, watching TV, or sleeping on the four day beds. The ladies left her alone; they seemed to understand, for they too had wandered the streets and alleys looking for comfort and a place to belong. Now Belle could begin her long journey back to herself.

NEAR PERFECT

Amy Haddad

Spun gold ringlets and blue eyes.
Chin quivering she softly repeats a mantra of "Mama, Mama"
as she moves to the corner of her hospital crib,
far from counterfeit mothers in white.

She jumps from the crib when Mama arrives.
Arms wrapped around her mother's neck,
legs around her waist.
All of the family is there,
father, grandparents, an aunt, a brother.
They stand in overalls and flannel,
white shoes and house dresses,
in awkward contrast to the
sterility and cleanliness of the room.

They all kiss her good-bye
as the cart comes to take her away,
watching as she disappears down the hall.
They wait in the doorway until the nurse tells
them to go to the surgical waiting room.
Dumbly, they move down the hallway,
grandparents, parents, aunt, and older brother.

She returns much later to the room,
limp and swaddled
with too many bandages for a biopsy.
Something is wrong, something is missing.
Her right arm is gone.

The muffled crying and anguish of her family
precede them down the hall.

They reach her room and for a moment there is silence,
then a collective gasp marking the reality of their loss
followed by a wail that rises,
crests, and fills the room.
She is alive, but she is not whole.
Her parents sob, "What will we do?"
"How could this happen to us?"
They bury their faces in their grief
and avoid the crib.

The child wakes,
taking in only her mother's face,
whimpers and reaches for her
not knowing her loss
or her parents' shame.

SPRING SEMESTER
Amy Haddad

"Brown, Ann—mother; Ruth—daughter; Jeffrey—son." I had found the clinical record that would be my introduction to one of the families I would care for in my community health rotation. Unlike other areas of nursing, where the patient comes to the professional, community health nursing requires visiting patients in their homes to get a more accurate picture of what the patient has to deal with on a daily basis. It's one thing to cope with a chronic medical problem or a new baby in the hospital, and quite another at home.

Once a week for the spring semester, I was to visit Ann, who was 30 years old, and her two children—Ruth, 8, and Jeffrey, 28 months. The clinical record was not very thick. The Brown family had only been admitted a week ago. I wanted to learn all I could before I went out to meet Ann and her children. Also, I was supposed to write a detailed plan of care for each member of the Brown household as part of the course requirements. My instructor had commented, "You can't really write a good care plan until you make your first visit. Even then you won't have the whole picture. Your care plan will never really be finished." Although this was somewhat discouraging, I began to jot notes as I read the history of Ann and her family.

Ann was schizophrenic. Although the term "chronic" had not been legitimized in mental health at the time, it certainly applied to Ann. She had been in and out of psychiatric hospitals since she was a teenager. All of the therapy—from electroconvulsive to drugs—had done little to change her psychosis except to keep it under wraps for a while until it would creep out again. Ann's personal history was sketchy. There was no information about her parents or childhood. No information about the man or men who fathered Ruth and Jeffrey. The only information I really got was that Ann had been released a few weeks ago from an inpatient psychiatric facility and would now be seen on an outpatient basis. The visiting nurse agency had been contacted to give her a weekly injection of fluphenazine or Prolixin—a long-acting antipsychotic drug. Ann was literally at the end of the antipsychotic road. There were no drugs any stronger at the time. My job would be to give Ann her weekly injection and check on her overall status.

The nurse who gave me the report on Ann said, "It's kind of good that we give this med to her IM. This way we're sure that she takes it and we have an excuse to check up on her and see how the kids are doing." Evidently, Ann could not be relied upon to take oral antipsychotic drugs, so the physicians had resorted to Prolixin.

A maxim of community health nursing is that the nurse takes care of the family, not just a single patient. So when Ann was referred to the visiting nurses, Ruth and Jeffrey automatically became patients as well. Ruth was in the second grade at a school two blocks from her home. There was no further information in the clinical record about Ruth. Jeffrey, however, provoked more interest. The record reflected concern about his numerous developmental delays—he didn't speak, wasn't toilet trained, couldn't use a cup.

I waited to make my first visit until late afternoon so Ruth would be home from school and I could see the whole family. I would be taking over the case from the regular visiting nurse, and so I needed to make a visit before the end of the week. Ann did not have a phone, so I had no way of calling and letting her know that I would be her nurse or what time I would be coming. I hoped they would be home.

Ann, Ruth, and Jeffrey lived in a two-story house that had been converted into four tiny apartments. I knocked on the door. As I waited I could hear a television in the background and a bright voice over the sound of the TV that said, "I'll get it." A little girl opened the door. She had short, straight dark brown hair. Her eyes were dark brown as well, and there was a sprinkling of freckles across her nose. She was wearing one of those flimsy, sleeveless cotton house dresses that snap down the front. It was a grown-up dress that had been cut and hemmed, rather badly, so it would not drag on the ground. The gaudy flower print was set off by several strands of variously colored beads looped around her neck. She looked like she had been playing dress-up.

The little girl leaned briefly on the door frame as she looked me up and down once. Before I could say a word, she said, "Mama's having a bad day. I'm Ruth. Don't talk loud or you'll wake up Gene and he gets awful mad. Do you want to see my brother? He's in the kitchen. So's Mama. What's your name? Be nice to Mama, she's having a bad day." All of this was spoken over her shoulder as she lead me back through the apartment to the kitchen.

On our way to the kitchen, out of the corner of my eye, I saw a man lying in a bed in one of the bedrooms. Even lying down he looked like a big man. This must be Gene, I thought. Gene was lying on his stomach, snoring, with his arms crossed above his head. He had a tattoo on the arm that I could just make out through the tangle of shoulder-length black hair that fell over his arms. I smelled a combination of vomit and whiskey as I walked by the bedroom.

Ruth said, "Mama, it's the nurse," as we turned into the kitchen.

Ann was leaning against the sink, smoking a cigarette with a great deal of difficulty. Her fingers and hands jerked rhythmically. Her upper lip trembled and she blinked in an irregular but continuous manner. She had her arms crossed and only uncrossed them to smoke. Even crossed, her hands and arms moved. In fact, she seemed to be in motion even though she was standing still. When she loosed the hand holding the cigarette, her arm would suddenly jerk up in a wide swing. It took her a great deal of effort to get the cigarette to her lips. The fingers of her right hand were yellowed from smoking. She took a long drag from the cigarette, recrossed her arms, started to take a few hesitant, shaky steps toward me, and said, "Hi," then sort of fell back against the kitchen counter.

Ann had on a white tee shirt with food stains down the front, jeans, and no shoes. Her hair was uncombed and dirty. I had not taken care of very many heavily medicated, psychotic patients, but Ann had the same look as others I had seen—dry, reddish skin and eyes that had the odd combination of being dull and startled simultaneously. She looked much older than thirty.

Jeffrey was sitting in a high chair. He was a chubby, curly-haired toddler. He was playing with food on his high chair tray. Like his mother, he had food down the front of his chest. He also had food all over his hands and in his hair. He was giggling and making little cooing sounds. He was naked except for double diapers. I could tell from my side of the kitchen that he needed to be changed.

"I'm a student nurse and I'm going to be taking care of you for the next few months," I began by way of introduction. "Could we sit down somewhere and talk?"

Ann led the way with shaky steps to a small table and two chairs. Ruth followed us and stood behind her mother and played with her necklaces.

I asked Ann, "How long have you had this shakiness?"

"Started two days ago," Ann replied.

"Has this happened before?"

"Sometimes, but not this bad."

I had seen a few patients react to antipsychotic drugs this way, but not this severely. At least I thought it was a reaction to the medication. Maybe Ann drank as well. I didn't know how to ask her if she did. I tried another approach.

"When did you get the first dose of your new medication?"

Ann looked blank.

I tried again. "You know, the shot the visiting nurse gave you after you got home from the hospital?"

Ruth answered, "She got it the day we had our pictures taken at school." Since Ruth could not remember the day her picture was taken, all I knew was that it was sometime last week.

I tried to complete at least some of the basic questions that I was supposed to ask about the general health of the children and Ann's status since her discharge. The whole time I was thinking about what I should do with Ann's next dose of medication. I was supposed to give her another shot of Prolixin. If the medication was causing her shakiness and I gave her the shot, I would make it worse. If it wasn't the medication and I didn't give her the shot, she might get psychotic. Furthermore, if I didn't give her the shot, I would have to explain withholding the medication to someone. At the least, I would have to explain it to my instructor. I had no idea what the drug's duration of action was, so I didn't know how quickly she might suffer from more severe side effects or go crazy.

I told Ann, "I need to go and call your doctor and let him know about this shakiness. I don't think you should be having this kind of problem. I'll be back in a few minutes."

Ruth followed me outside and watched as I walked a block up to the corner to a pay phone and called my instructor and explained what I had seen. She said, "You'll have to call her physician." I called her physician at the clinic and amazingly got to speak to him. I went through my explanation again. He was not very familiar with Ann and said as much. He told me to give her the injection and to have her come into the clinic the next day so he could take a look at her. He hung up before I could ask him if giving her the shot would make things worse.

I walked back to Ann's house. Ruth was still standing outside. I followed her back into the house and quietly shied past the still-slumbering Gene to the kitchen. Ann had not moved from the little kitchen table. I hesitated as I said, "The doctor says you should get your medicine and come and see him at the clinic tomorrow." Ann didn't say anything, but she stood up very carefully and held on to the counter. She stepped sideways with her back to me and moved down the counter closer to where I was standing. She leaned forward and with great effort unbuttoned and unzipped her jeans. She reached around and pulled down her jeans and underpants so that her left cheek was exposed. The whole time she was doing this I did not have a clue that she was getting ready for me to give her the shot. I don't know where I thought I was going to give her this injection, but the kitchen wasn't what I expected. I hadn't even washed my hands, yet here she was holding on to the counter with one hand so she wouldn't fall and holding her pants down with the other.

I was embarrassed for her. I could feel my face burn. How humiliating to stand here in the kitchen so exposed, so trusting. I was afraid she might fall, so I quickly got out the medication and syringe. Prior to this, I had had all the time in the world to draw up medication for injection. Now I felt as if I should do it quickly, even though Ann said nothing. My hands shook as I drew it up and gave her the shot.

As Ann was fastening her pants she said, "I don't know how I'm going to get to the doctor's. I don't think I can walk to the bus stop."

"I'll take you," I said without thinking. "I'll get you at two tomorrow." I left before Gene could wake up.

The next morning my instructor was horrified when she learned that I had volunteered to take Ann to the clinic.

"How do you think she will manage this kind of problem when you aren't there to solve it for her?" she said. "She'll have to take a cab. Call her case worker for a voucher."

I hadn't thought about what Ann would do in the future. I was worried about today. Chastened, I got the taxi voucher and went to Ann's. On the way there I wondered if I should have gotten the voucher for Ann or if I should have made her get it. I gave her the voucher. We walked to the corner to call the cab. I helped her dial the cab company. I wrote out instructions about how to find the doctor's office once she got to the clinic. I waited with her at the door until I saw the cab. It was not until Ann was pulling away in the cab that I realized Jeffrey was alone in the apartment taking his nap. How could I have forgotten him? How could Ann forget him? Did she just expect that I would take care of him? But how? I was locked out of the apartment and he was alone inside. I walked around the building but could see no way in other than breaking a window. No one else answered their buzzer to let me in the building. Even if I could have gotten into the building, I didn't have a key to the apartment.

Not knowing what else to do, I sat on the front steps and waited for Ann to come back from the doctor or Ruth to come home from school. I fluctuated between anger, fear, and frustration as I waited. The image of the Duchess's fish footman in *Alice in Wonderland* came to mind as I sat there, like him, staring stupidly up at the sky. "I shall sit here," the footman remarked, "till tomorrow—or the next day, maybe." I knew how the footman felt. Unlike the constant howling and sneezing going on inside the Duchess's house in *Alice*, there was only the occasional passing car to break the silence. I could have sat in my car to keep warm, but I was afraid to move that far away from Jeffrey, as if my presence on the porch would somehow keep him safe, somehow comfort him if he woke from his nap.

Finally, Ruth's small brown head bobbed just above a hedge as she made her way up the sidewalk.

"What are you doing here?" she asked. "Why are you sitting on the stoop?"

"Your mom's at the doctor and I'm watching your brother."

"Out here?" she persisted.

"I got locked out."

Ruth fished a key out of her pocket and opened the door. Jeffrey was wet but otherwise fine. I changed him and decided to give him a bath. Ruth watched and told me about school— who her teacher was, what she had learned. When I had Jeffrey cleaned and dressed, Ruth said to Jeffrey, "It's time to eat, kiddo."

I followed her to the kitchen and watched as she made their supper. She got bologna and cheese slices, Miracle Whip, and a jar of applesauce from the refrigerator. She had to make another trip for the milk. She got some paper plates and proceeded to make sandwiches for herself and her brother.

"I like Miracle Whip on my sandwich, but Jeffrey likes his plain," she said by way of explanation as she placed bread, cheese, and meat on her brother's plate. She spooned out some applesauce onto each plate.

"Can I help?" I asked.

"Could we have some alphabet soup? I'm not to use the stove, but you could. It's right up in the cupboard."

She got a saucepan out while I got the soup down from the shelf.

"Where's the can opener?" I asked.

She handed me a key-type manual can opener from the drawer. I had only used an electric can opener. I tried to figure out how the manual can opener worked. Ruth watched me for a few minutes then said, "I know how it works," and opened the can.

I watched Ruth and Jeffrey eat and restrained myself from feeding Jeffrey to keep him clean. He managed to eat what he wanted then proceeded to play with what was left. Ruth said, "I sure love this soup. Look at all the letters."

Ruth and I cleaned up the kitchen. I felt guilty about everything I did. Even the simple act of washing the dishes seemed suspect. I could hear my instructor's voice warning me about encouraging dependency, taking on roles that weren't mine.

At 6:45, Ann finally pulled up in a cab. I was angry and frantic. I had begun to think that she might not come back.

"Ann, what took you so long? I can't watch your children like this. I'm not supposed to. What would you have done if I hadn't been here?" I asked.

Ann looked confused, then said, "Ruth takes care of Jeffrey when I'm gone."

I never told anyone that Ann left her children alone. I was afraid someone would take them away from her if they knew.

I visited once a week until May. The ambitious goals I had set for Ann and her family were reduced to trying to toilet train Jeffrey and control the side effects of Ann's medication. Strangely, these two tasks were tied together. Ann couldn't get Jeffrey to the potty chair in time because she could barely walk and move herself. Once I was able to get the physician to order Cogentin, a drug to manage the neuromuscular side effects of the Prolixin, Ann could move without shaking.

"Another nurse will be seeing you instead of me," I told Ann during my last visit.

"Okay," she responded. There was no emotion on her part. Just another of numerous adjustments to outsiders in her life.

But Ruth followed me outside as she had on my first visit. "Here," she said and handed me a wallet-size copy of her school picture—a beaming smile, freckles, flowered house dress, and beads. "So you remember me."

UNIVERSAL PRECAUTIONS

Veneta Masson

It's wearing gloves mainly,
like the ambulance driver
who came to take you away.
He had on a pair when he slammed through the door
but when he saw you there
bleeding and heaving
he pulled out another
from a bulging back pocket
and snapped them on
over the first—
one pair for protocol
one pair for fear.

If all it takes
for peace of mind
is a layer of latex
then I say why not—
and why?

TOBACCO, TULIPS, AND TERMINAL CARE

Maryella Desak Sirmon

Seventy-two hours was a long time. But soon the conflicts would be resolved. While John's body struggled for breath and his soul struggled for eternity, she considered the internal conflict she faced. What role should she play? Doctor? Daughter? Could she somehow be both? As she contemplated his death, memories of his life and their shared bonds trickled in. She reached across and held his hand and automatically checked a redial pulse for rate and rhythm.

John smoked—a lot. Mostly back when cigarettes and martinis were still fashionable and Ronald Reagan's face adorned Chesterfield posters. Early years on the farm that his immigrant father had dug out of the Pennsylvania countryside were filled with responsibility and love. Childhood dreams were born in a one-room clapboard schoolhouse with eight grades huddled around a coal stove. The teacher, fresh from the Pennsylvania Normal School, gave John his first taste of books and cigarettes. Neither one seemed dangerous at the time.

Then came that special girl. But her matriarchal Southern mother did not approve of the damn Yankee. Although she banished him from her house and her daughter, she could not stop the letters and the secret meetings. Soon the two young lovers stole away to the church up the street, picking up the required witnesses along the way. There they etched their love into the county registrar's book and eventually into the old lady's family Bible.

With Pearl Harbor, life settled into a happy routine of marriage, postponed dreams, and ration books that doled out cigarettes and sugar. Postwar days saw a good job as a machinist, promotion to shop foreman, a new baby girl, and a sense that some dreams could come true. Then came the angel of sudden death for his beloved wife. Her progressive mitral stenosis from old rheumatic disease brought her to the university hospital for one of the first commissurotomies, but not soon enough. At forty-six, he was left with his daughter, his books, and his Camels.

His world now centered on this little girl, who was both the remnant of his love and his life. He moved next door to the big white-columned house of his mother-in-law. There she and two widowed daughters, who had returned to the only home they had left, carefully watched over the child. Yes, there were days the little girl missed the presence of a woman she barely knew. But most days she was far too busy growing up in the safety of a father's love to be disturbed by such things.

As she grew, she shared John's passion for books and listened with her heart as he taught her compassion and integrity. School passed quickly and easily. She basked in his paternal pride. Then she declared her intention to apply to medical school. The family told her that Marcus Welby was a figment of some television producer's vivid imagination. But her father's piercing blue eyes just smiled. He reassured her that sensitivity and science were not mutually exclusive. Armed with his confidence and the innocent courage of youth, she soon conquered medical school, residency, and fellowship, and returned home to the university. The relationship with her father changed. Although John could never quite relinquish his little-girl picture of her, they now talked as adults. During long hours over coffee, they shared ideas. With her support he had quit smoking during her medical school years. But this decision had come too late.

Caring for him as a daughter and not a physician, she entrusted him to Dr. Mike, her favorite pulmonologist. This triangle worked well. John continued a restricted but independent life in his own home, enjoying frequent visits from his two young grandsons. During these years, her career matured uneventfully until she was asked to assume the position of course master for the ethics program in the medical school. Without hesitation, she said yes. She had always been interested in ethics and she eagerly greeted this challenge. Fearing some inadequacy that might hamper her students, she immediately enrolled in graduate coursework in bioethics and returned again to the books that she had always loved. To enrich the offerings, she brought in physicians and ethicists of different backgrounds to work with the courses. The students met her enthusiasm in kind, and as students always do if allowed, taught her. Soon her work expanded to include house staff education and often faculty as well. The problems were rarely easy and often none of the alternatives were pleasing.

Then the tobacco years began to catch up with John. The baseball games with his grandsons were replaced by checkers. The pulmonary function test results and arterial blood gases began their slow downward spiral. Finally, Dr. Mike suggested gently that now was the time for home oxygen. John was skeptical and reluctant to encumber what little freedom he had left, but was soon persuaded by the relentless dyspnea that dogged his every step. He asked her, "What do you think?" She hedged, "That's what we have Dr. Mike for." The Gemini twins of doctor and daughter battled to an uneasy truce. She arranged to be at his home when they delivered the system—a compressor for the house and a large liquid tank to refill the portable canister. She listened closely as they educated father and daughter about how it all worked.

John adapted quickly to his new appendage, and it could be found trailing him up a ladder as he hung new curtains in his house or under his car as he changed the oil. None of her elegant persuasion could slow him down. "So what if I fall off the ladder and break a hip? Maybe I'll die quickly," he would say. Only his worsening dyspnea could slow him.

Then one Thanksgiving, John made his first of many journeys to the medical intensive care unit. The careful attention of Dr. Mike and the house staff paid off and John slid home, bypassing any real consideration of a ventilator. Three months and three hospitalizations later, John and his daughter sat in his room talking when one of her favorite residents came in.

"You know, I think I would like to take a trip," John said.

Not sure where this was leading, the resident replied, "Oh?"

"Yes, to Holland," said John.

The resident shifted his weight on uncomfortable feet and said, "That would be nice. I believe the tulips there are really beautiful."

"Maybe," said John. "But mostly I would like Holland because they let you put people to sleep there, like we do animals when they're suffering."

The resident's eyes mirrored the apprehension that crept into his soul. He rambled on about how John was a long way from that. The older man just smiled. His daughter, the doctor, thought a long time about what he had said.

John went home, calm and stable again for a time. Then Dr. Mike called: "John has discussed suicide with me and has made specific plans. I think you'd better remove the guns in his house if you can without upsetting him." Her father had collected and rebuilt antique firearms for many years. His finest pieces were displayed in a gun case he had carved by hand. And so, when John was away playing with his grandsons, she arranged to have all the ammunition and firing pins removed and stored in her house. If John ever noticed, he never spoke of their absence.

Another month, another hospitalization. Again he cheated the ventilator and made it to the floor. Then early one morning, her phone rang. John appeared to be in respiratory failure and in imminent danger of arresting. The resident had already called Dr. Mike. Dutifully noting the do-not-resuscitate order on the chart, the resident wanted to verify its accuracy.

"Yes, that's correct," she said. "If he arrests, you are not to begin CPR. You may go with inhaled beta agonists and other meds, but no intubation. I'm on my way." Her calm voice masked the terror she felt in her heart at losing this special person. She drove slowly and deliberately; a selfish part of her wished he would be gone before she arrived, sparing her the inevitable. He was not. The medicines had worked their magic again.

Two more months and two more hospitalizations later, she continued to think. Home was no longer an option. After his last discharge, she had arranged around-the-clock sitters. John stayed at home less than twenty-four hours. Whether from hypoxia or the blessing of some unseen angel, John became more forgetful and understood fewer details around him. After thoughtful consideration, she chose a hospice program especially known for its respiratory care. It was a hard choice, one made with her memory of his previous wishes and not his mind now. Dr. David, the director, was both a geriatrician and a treasured friend of many years. The staff were efficient, caring, and concerned beyond her expectations, but that could not stop the tears as she toured the facility. Her promise of professional detachment withered and died.

The days and weeks stretched into spring and early summer, and she almost believed John could get well and go home. Dr. David mercifully said no. She came daily. John enjoyed the garden, where she often took him to sit. They talked, reminisced, and tried desperately to hold fast to the moment.

Then came the yellow sputum again. The well-balanced triangle was now without one of its points, so the two remaining decided to forego the hospital and parenteral antibiotics and a ventilator in favor of oral antibiotics and continued close attention to respiratory therapy. Without speaking it, they knew what this would mean. She telephoned her office to cancel outpatients and lectures for the next several days. Fortunately, she was not on service; her partners had already accommodated her father's illness many times and she was glad she would not have to ask yet another time. The students had just turned in their final exams from the introductory ethics course, and she carried those to his bedside as she sat and they talked and waited together.

As the hours passed, John talked less and she thought more. The questions she graded took on a haunting significance: define and give an example of microallocation and macroallocation of health care; should health care for the elderly be limited—why or why not; develop two arguments for or against physician-assisted suicide; is physician participation in active euthanasia compatible with the practice of medicine in today's world and justify your answer; contrast three differences between the traditional Hippocratic oath and any one of the modern versions studied in class. She though of Quintan and Brophy and Cruzan, of Debbie and her ovarian cancer, and especially of Diane and Dr. Quill and the covenants that bind parent to child and physician to patient.

Seventy-two hours was a very long time. In the papers she held, innocent young students argued the pros and cons of assisted suicide and euthanasia. Before her eyes, John struggled and fought for every breath. In her mind, she saw tulips and heard the echoes of his wish for a trip to Holland. In her heart, she cried and wished for the courage to act.

Would it be so wrong to use the skills he had encouraged her to gain? The battling forces she faced were not good and evil, but rather the little girl who loved her daddy and wanted to stop his suffering, and the trained physician who wondered if medicine has the right to assert absolute control over every process of life. The decision to withhold John's care was a definable act with both an intent and a soon-to-be-seen effect. A syringe of stolen morphine, easily obtained and used compassionately, would also have intent and effect. Could she truly say that between these two acts there existed a moral difference of such magnitude that the scene before her was justified? In the end, she was powerless against the person he had taught her to be. When the time came, she quietly held him in her arms and kissed him good-bye. Then she rang for the nurse: "My father just died. The time was 3:49 A.M."

(first appeared in *Annals of Internal Medicine,* vol. 119, no. 10 [November 1993])

UNTITLED (HAIKU)

Susan Ogborn

"Problem is," he gasped,
"communication." I am
crushed at our failures.

Contributors' Biographies

KATE BROWN combines medical anthropology and ethics as an associate professor in Creighton University's Center for Health Policy and Ethics and School of Pharmacy and Allied Health Professions. She uses creative writing, literary interpretation, and theater in her teaching. She publishes across disciplines in the fields of culture, bioethics, and health policy. She is cofounder of a writing group and is an editorial board member of the Literature, Arts, and Medicine Database (http://endeavor. med.nyu.edu). Her Ph.D., in sociomedical sciences, is from Columbia University.

CORTNEY DAVIS, a nurse practitioner, is the author of *The Body Flute* (Adastra Press, 1994) and *Details of the Flesh* (Calyx Books, 1997), and coeditor of *Between the Heartbeats: Poetry and Prose by Nurses* (University of Iowa Press, 1995). Her poems have appeared in the *Hudson Review, Poet & Critic, Journal of the American Medical Association, Literature and Medicine, Yankee, Calyx*, and other journals. She received an NEA grant in poetry and two Connecticut Commission on the Arts grants.

KIM DAYTON is a professor of law at the University of Kansas, where she teaches courses in feminist theory, civil and criminal procedures, and the law of cyberspace. She frequently uses legal texts and narrative and literary works in her classes to explore bioethical issues of special concern to women.

AMY HADDAD is a registered nurse who specializes in ethics education in the health sciences. She has published several books and numerous journal articles in the area of ethics and clinical practice in a variety of health disciplines. Her poems have been published in the *American Journal of Nursing, Fetishes* (University of Colorado Health Sciences), and *Between the Heartbeats* (University of Iowa Press, 1995). She is a professor in the Center for Health Policy and Ethics and the School of Pharmacy and Allied Health Professions at Creighton University.

BARBARA JESSING is a family and child therapist with Family Service in Omaha, Nebraska. Her interests include the therapeutic uses of writing by practitioners and their clients. Her work has been published in the anthology *Leaning into the Wind: Women Write from the Heart of the West* (Houghton Mifflin, 1997) and in the journal *Fine Lines*.

VENETA MASSON is a family nurse practitioner as well as a poet and essayist. Her chapbook, *Just Who*, from which some of her poetry is taken, is a collection of poems and photographs from the life of a small inner-city clinic in Washington, D.C. A new collection of poetry, *Rehab at the Florida Avenue Grill*, is forthcoming.

SUSAN OGBORN is currently the director of education for the Greater Omaha Chamber of Commerce. Previously, she was director of Human Resources and Quality Management for University Hospital at the University of Nebraska Medical Center. She has published numerous articles in health care journals and in education publications.

KELLY JENNINGS OLSON earned her master's degree in English and creative writing from the University of Nebraska-Lincoln and her bachelor's degree from Augustana College. Her stories have appeared in *Laurus* and the *St. Anthony Messenger*. A former volunteer emergency medical technician on a small-town ambulance crew, she now freelances as a writer and graphic designer.

CLAUDIA PEYTON is an assistant professor and the chair of the Department of Occupational Therapy at Creighton University. She is a graduate of the University of Southern California and Loma Linda University. Her publications focus on the theory and practice of neuro-occupation.

RUTH PURTILO is a physical therapist and professor of ethics. She is the director of the Center for Health Policy and Ethics at Creighton University and teaches ethics in the medical school. She has published professionally in health-professions journals and is the author of two ethics textbooks. She earned her master's and Ph.D. degrees from Harvard University.

JUDY HOPKINS SCHAEFER, a hemophilia nurse specialist and part-time faculty member at the Pennsylvania State University, is the author of *Harvesting the Dew* (Vista, 1997), and is coeditor of the first international anthology of creative writing by nurses, *Between the Heartbeats* (University of Iowa Press, 1995). She is coordinator of the Poetry Department and the *American Journal of Nursing* and is active with two medically related journals, *Wild Onions* and *Mediphors*.

AUDREY SHAFER is an associate professor of anesthesiology at Stanford University and the Veterans Administration Palo Alto Health Care System. She teaches several medical humanities courses, including a literature and medicine course for medical students, and has published poetry in medical and literary journals.

MARYELLA DESAK SIRMON is a physician and writer living in Mobile, Alabama. Her special interests are medical ethics and the art of medicine. A nephrologist, she is an associate professor at the University of Southern Alabama, College of Medicine, where she received her M.D. degree. She completed postgraduate training at the University of Alabama at Birmingham, Duke University Medical Center, and Georgetown University.

RUTH ANN VOGEL, a retired school nurse, resides in Stanton, Nebraska. She is a graduate of the University of Nebraska College of Nursing. In recent years she has won second and third place and honorable mentions in the State Chaparral Poetry Contests. Her poems appear in *Midwest Poetry Review* and in *Gold Words*, an anthology of winners by senior poets.

SISTER CASHEL WEILER has a B.S.N. from St. Teresa's College and a master's degree in health administration from the University of Minnesota. She works in critical care medical research for the MAYO Medical Center in Rochester, Minnesota. She has published professionally in medical, nursing, hospital, and business journals. Her poems are published in *Womenpsalms* (Saint Mary's Press, Christian Brothers Publication) and in *Image: Journal of Nursing Scholarship*.

LYNNE WILLETT is a pediatrician in Omaha, Nebraska, whose special interest is medical ethics. She has published many scientific articles but enjoys writing freelance to manage stress. She graduated from the University of Nebraska College of Medicine, and her clinical specialty is neonatology.

Books of Related Interest

Reconstructing Illness
Studies in Pathology, Second Edition

by Anne Hunsaker Hawkins

This second edition includes a thoroughly revised and expanded appendix and a new chapter on the myths of self-narrative and ethical concerns.

Recommended for medical practitioners, the clergy, caregivers, students of popular culture, and the general reader, *Reconstructing Illness* demonstrates that "only when we hear both the doctor's and the patient's voice will we have a medicine that is truly human."

> *"The book has earned an important place in courses on medical practice as well as courses treating any of the various relationships between story and healing and is accessible and engaging enough to be useful to all who struggle with serious illness."*— Medical Humanities Review

1999
289 pages
6 × 9
ISBN 1-55753-126-9
Paper $18.95

Published by
Purdue University Press

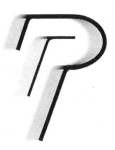

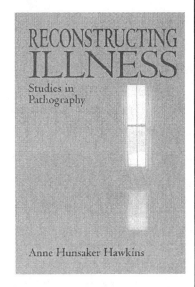

RECONSTRUCTING
ILLNESS
Studies in
Pathography

Anne Hunsaker Hawkins

Books of Related Interest

The Complete Guide to Alzheimer's-Proofing Your Home

by Mark Warner, Ageless Design

Written by a practicing architect and gerontologist, *The Complete Guide to Alzheimer's-Proofing Your Home* shows you how to create a home environment that will help you cope with the many difficulties associated with Alzheimer's disease. This unique book is divided into two sections to provide the most thorough coverage available. Section One deals with interior and exterior spaces individually, providing key information on how to ensure that the Alzheimer's patient will be safe and secure. Section Two gives a detailed list of potential problems related to Alzheimer's and practical information on how to cope with those problems in the home setting.

> "... *comprehensive coverage of the specifics of caring for afflicted loved ones in the home. A superlative resource for home caregivers.*"—Booklist

1998
470 pages
7 × 10
ISBN 1-55753-127-7
Cloth $29.95

Published by
Purdue University Press

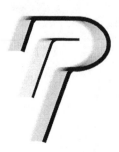

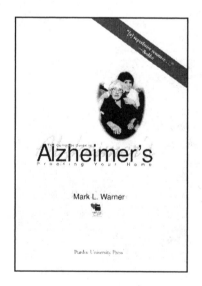